Glucagon in Gastroenterology

Glucagon
in Gastroenterology

Edited by J. Picazo, M.D.

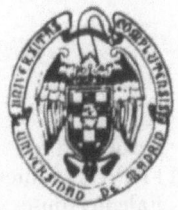

The Proceedings of an International Workshop held in Madrid on 31 May 1978 under the auspices of the Medical School of the Universidad Complutense, Madrid.

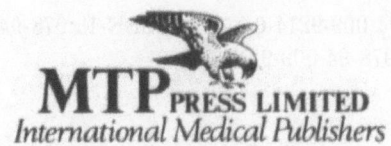

MTP PRESS LIMITED
International Medical Publishers

Published by
MTP Press Limited
Falcon House
Lancaster, England

Copyright © 1979 MTP Press Limited
Softcover reprint of the hardcover 1st edition 1979

ISBN-13:978-94-009-9214-6   e-ISBN-13:978-94-009-9212-2
DOI: 10.1007/978-94-009-9212-2

Phototypesetting by Rainbow Graphics, Liverpool

Contents

List of Participants

A.L. Baker
Department of Medicine
University of Chicago
Chicago, IL 60637
USA

B. Ek
Section of Gastroenterology
Department of Medicine
University of Umeå
Umeå
Sweden

A. Gomez-Pan
Department of Experimental
Endocrinology
Medical School of the
Universidad Complutense
Madrid
Spain

J.B. Jaspan
Department of Medicine
Section of Endocrinology
University of Chicago
Chicago, IL 60637
USA

L. Kreel
Division of Radiology
Clinical Research Centre and
Northwick Park Hospital
Harrow HA1 3UJ
United Kingdom

J.D. McCarthy
Department of Surgery
University of New Mexico
School of Medicine
Albuquerque, NM 87123
USA

J. Myren
Department of Gastroenterology
Ullevål Hospital
Oslo 1
Norway

F. Paul
Centre of Internal Medicine
Justus Liebig University
Giessen
West Germany

E. Pearce
*The London Hospital Medical
    College
Academic Unit of Gastroenterology
The London Hospital
London E1 1BB
United Kingdom*

M.-J. Treffot
*Hôpital La Conception
Centre de Gastroentérologie
Marseille
France*

N.A. Volpicelli
*Gastrointestinal Section
Lovelace Medical Center
Albuquerque, NM 87123
USA*

D.L. Wingate
*The London Hospital Medical
    College
Academic Unit of Gastroenterology
The London Hospital
London E1 1BB
United Kingdom*

Preface

It was with very much pleasure that I accepted the invitation to chair this workshop on *Glucagon in Gastroenterology*. Not least among the reasons for my accepting was the fact that it would get me out from behind my administrator's desk at the university and enable me to spend what promised to be a few refreshing hours in a field where so much is apparently happening.

Another reason for my accepting was the attractiveness of the format planned for the workshop. It was to be a *working* event. The programme had been carefully planned to ensure that all aspects of the subject were covered and a very tight schedule was drawn up for we had to deal with the whole field in just one day. There was to be a small, truly international, list of participants, and, apart from those presenting papers, only two or three specially invited observers were to be present. Above all, perhaps, was the fact that the meeting was to be a multi-disciplinary one. This final point did indeed prove to be an extremely valuable one, for, as one of the participants remarked towards the end of the meeting: 'We all work busily away in our own particular fields, but to a large extent it is only when we are brought away and introduced to people working in other fields, and find, to our surprise, that they are working on the same things as us, that we know what the problems really are.'

The workshop took place in Madrid on 31st May 1978. The papers presented are published in this book, together with edited versions of the discussions which followed each presentation. Two exceptions occur, in that there is no discussion after the paper of Dr Gomez-Pan nor after that of Dr Treffot. I have to explain that, in the first case, Dr Gomez-Pan stepped into the

9

breach at literally overnight notice to take the place of the scheduled speaker who was unable to attend. The discussion which followed his presentation was not really pertinent to the paper which he subsequently wrote for publication, and so is not included. As far as Dr Treffot is concerned, at the very last minute she too was unfortunately unable to travel to Madrid. Her paper was read to the meeting, but, as the author was not present to answer questions, no real discussion was possible.

As chairman of the workshop I had far less work to do than anyone else, which is another appealing aspect of being chairman. One thing I am allowed to do though is to extend the thanks, and this I gladly do. First of all, and most sincerely, I thank all those who came to Madrid to participate in this workshop, both those who presented papers, and those who gave us the benefit of their opinions and experience during the discussion sessions. My thanks are also extended to Dr José Picazo and to Pamela Freebody who gathered all the material together, edited the discussions, and arranged for the publication of this book, and to Dr D.R. Owens for his assistance and helpful criticism in the editing process. Finally, and most especially, they are extended to Dr John Mumford of Novo Industri A/S, Denmark, who arranged for his company to organize and sponsor the whole event.

A. Oriol Bosch
Dean, Madrid Universidad
Complutense, Medical School

1 Glucagon as a Drug

A. Gomez-Pan, G. Blesa Malpica, M.D. Rodriguez Arnao and A. Oriol Bosch

The importance of glucagon as a hormone involved in nutrient homeostasis is rapidly growing. Its role in physiology and pathophysiology has recently been the subject of some excellent reviews.[1-4] In addition, however, glucagon has a number of pharmacological properties which are not necessarily related to its physiological role. A review of the clinical applications of glucagon as a drug forms the basis of this introductory chapter.

ACTIONS ON GROWTH HORMONE SECRETION

Roth and his co-workers first reported in 1963 that the administration of glucagon is followed by a rise in plasma growth hormone (GH) levels.[5] At that time the mechanism of glucagon-induced GH release was a rather controversial issue. The rise in GH levels was thought to be due to the stress of nausea often caused by glucagon,[6] but this seems unlikely since not all responders become nauseated after the injection. Most authors now accept that the release of GH after glucagon is independent of the blood sugar changes,[7 8] but some argue that a fall in blood glucose levels after the initial rise is essential for a positive GH response.[9] Mitchell and his colleagues[10] described a test for assessing GH reserve by administering 1 mg of glucagon subcutaneously and blood sampling for GH and glucose estimations both before and at intervals for 3 h afterwards. Normal subjects are expected to exceed basal GH levels by at least 6 ng/ml/3 h post glucagon. Cain et al.,[11] trying various routes of administration, found the subcutaneous test to be the most reliable. In their hands the glucagon test yielded less false negative results than the infusion of arginine, but was not as reliable as the insulin tolerance test. The glucagon stimulation test offers a good alternative for assessing pituitary GH reserve in those cases in which the performance of insulin-induced hypoglycaemia is contraindicated. Beta-adrenergic blockade enhances the GH releasing efficacy of glucagon. Concomitant administration of propranolol and glucagon results in less false negative results and renders the test more reliable.[12] [13]

ACTIONS ON CATECHOLAMINE SECRETION

Glucagon stimulates catecholamine release from the adrenal medulla and this effect is more marked in patients harbouring a phaeochromocytoma. Lefèbvre *et al.*[14] reported a case of a patient with a phaeochromocytoma in whom intravenous administration of 1 mg glucagon was followed by an abrupt release of catecholamines and a pressor response. This effect was not clinically significant after surgical excision of the tumour. The pressor response to intravenous administration of 0.5–1 mg glucagon has been successfully used as a diagnostic test for phaeochromocytoma[15-17] but experience so far is limited. The most reliable tests for the diagnosis of phaeochromocytoma, however, both in terms of safety and of accuracy, are those based on urinary catecholamine excretion. Glucagon has a definite place as a pharmacological test when standard methods of diagnosis yield conflicting results. It is safer than the tyramine, histamine, or phentolamine tests, but it is not free from unwanted effects, as it can produce a severe hypertensive response in patients with phaeochromocytoma.

GLUCAGON AS A TOOL IN LIVER FUNCTION TESTS

The physiological stimulus of glucagon on hepatic glycogenolysis has been used to assess liver function. Administration of glucagon to normal individuals is followed by an early rise in blood glucose of at least 50% above basal levels. Patients with hepatic cirrhosis exhibit a blunted response.[18] [19] This diagnostic test is also of value for the diagnosis of glycogen storage diseases.

The increase of circulating levels of cyclic adenosine

monophosphate (cAMP) induced by glucagon[20] has been shown to be due to an action at a hepatic level.[21][22] Davies *et al.*[2] showed that intravenous administration of 1 mg of glucagon results in a rise in plasma concentration of cAMP, and that this rise is the same in patients with hepatic cirrhosis or with intrahepatic cholestasis as in normal subjects; patients with extrahepatic obstructions, however, show an exaggerated response. They concluded that this procedure may, therefore, be of value in the differential diagnosis of intra and extra hepatic obstructive jaundice and so an aid when deciding on the surgical procedure. Further work is required before glucagon can be assigned a definite place as a tool to investigate liver function.

ACTIONS ON GASTRIC ACID SECRETION

Insulin-induced hypoglycaemia has long been known to stimulate gastric acid secretion via vagal stimulation and it is now a routine gastric secretory test in the intact animal. Early observations indicated that during this test the expected stimulation of gastric acid output was preceded by a transient inhibition of gastric acidity. This was thought to be due to the reactive hyperglucagonaemia induced by insulin hypo-glycaemia. Quirarte *et al.*,[24] showed that glucagon is a potent inhibitor of gastric acid secretion. It has recently been shown that the inhibition of gastric secretion by glucagon is due to a direct effect and cannot be abolished by alpha- or beta-adrenergic blockade.[25]

Gastric hyperacidity is a common feature in newborn babies[26] and has been shown to be due to gastrin hypersecretion.[27] This hypersecretory state declines gradually after the second day of life in spite of persistent high plasma gastrin concentrations, and the reduced gastric acid output has been attributed to elevated glucagon levels.[27] This report lends further support to the concept of glucagon acting directly on the parietal cell.

Konturek and co-workers[28] have shown that glucagon inhibits gastric acid and pepsin secretion in patients with duodenal ulcers, both basally and in response to a meal or pentagastrin. This inhibition is dose dependent. Histamine-induced gastric secretion is only slightly (though significantly) reduced by glucagon. Somatostatin, a potent inhibitor of gastric acid and pepsin secretion[29] has a very similar pattern of inhibition to that of glucagon.[30] It has been shown that glucagon stimulates somatostatin release.[31] Whether glucagon inhibits gastric secretion directly or via somatostatin has not yet been elucidated.

The clinical applications of glucagon as an inhibitor of gastric acid secretion in patients with duodenal ulcers or the Zollinger–Ellison syndrome require further study. The availability of histamine-2 receptor antagonists for routine clinical use lessen the need for glucagon in this field, but an analogue with preferential effects on the stomach, and negligible hyperglycaemic action, would clearly be of value.

ACTIONS ON CARDIAC CONTRACTILITY

Glucagon has intrinsic inotropic and chronotropic effects on the heart.[32] It increases the velocity of atrioventricular conduction, but has no effect on ventricular automaticity.[33] The enhancement of sinus activity combined with a lack of effect on Purkinje fibres facilitates the antiarrhythmic action of glucagon.[33-36] Brogan *et al.*[37] successfully treated a group of patients with congestive cardiac failure who had failed to respond to conventional therapy. Similarly encouraging results have been reported by several other groups.[38-42] The use of glucagon or of one of its analogues in the treatment of cardiac failure, when routine methods have not been successful, is clearly indicated.

METABOLIC EFFECTS

(i) **Hyperglycaemia**

Glucagon produces a hyperglycaemic effect in the presence of normal glycogen stores when given subcutaneously, intramuscularly, or intravenously. In healthy subjects the blood glucose level rises by 30–90 mg/100 ml, 20–30 min after the injection.

Glucagon has frequently been used in the treatment of severe insulin-induced hypoglycaemia in diabetic patients when oral or intravenous administration of glucose was not possible.[43] The usual dosage is 1 mg intramuscularly. The advantage of glucagon over glucose administration in the treatment of severe hypoglycaemia is that glucagon can be easily and effectively administered to the unconscious patient. It can restore normoglycaemia within 10 minutes, and maintain blood sugar levels in the normal range for over an hour, allowing time for the oral administration of glucose.

(ii) **Hypoglycaemia**

Glucagon stimulates insulin secretion from the alpha cells of the pancreas by a direct action. It promotes acute insulin release and hepatic glycogenolysis.

It can be used as a provocative test for insulin hypersecretion. The blood glucose and plasma insulin response may be helpful in the differential diagnosis of fasting hypoglycaemia.[44] After an overnight fast, glucagon (30 μg/kg to a maximum of 1 mg) is injected intravenously over 2 min, or intramuscularly, and samples obtained for glucose and insulin at 0, 2, 5, 10, 15, 30, 45, 60, 90 and 120 min. If an excessive insulin response is found within the first few minutes of the parenteral glucagon, islet cell hyperfunction is probable. It may be associated with a subnormal rise in blood glucose or even with a reactive hypoglycaemia.[45] A blunted glucose response with a normal insulin rise indicates hepatic or other endocrine organ dysfunction in the genesis of the hypoglycaemia. In healthy subjects the plasma insulin concentration rises rapidly to reach a peak of 30–100 mU/1 above the baseline values 5–10 minutes after the glucagon injection, and usually returns to the baseline within 20–60 mins.[46]

CONCLUDING COMMENTS

In this paper an effort has been made to analyze the possible therapeutic applications of glucagon. It is acknowledged that some of the actions described may well be merely pharmacological and have no physiological relevance at all. In addition to the well-established properties briefly reviewed here, glucagon has a number of other important pharmacological actions. Some of these are dealt with in other contributions to this workshop; others are at an experimental stage and require further investigation before being tested in man.

Acknowledgement

The authors wish to thank Ms. Joan E. Mutchnick for her excellent secretarial assistance in the preparation of this paper.

References

1 Marks, V. (1972). Glucagon. *Clin. Endocrinol. Metab.*, **3**, 829.
2 Sherwing, R. and Felig, P. (1977). New concepts in glucagon physiology. In P. P. Foa, J. S. Bajaj, and N. L. Foa (eds.) *Glucagon: Its Role in Physiology and Clinical Medicine*, p.595 (New York: Springer-Verlag).
3 Unger, R. H., Raskin, P., Srikant, C. B. and Orci, L. (1977). Glucagon and the A cells. In R. O. Greep (ed.) *Recent Progress in Hormone Research*, vol. 33, p. 477 (New York: Academic Press).
4 Gerich, J. E. and Lorenzi, M. (1978). The role of the autonomic nervous system and somatostatin in the control of insulin and glucagon secretion. In W. F. Ganong and L. Martini (eds.) *Frontiers of Neuroendocrinology*, vol. 5, p. 265 (New York: Raven Press).
5 Roth, J., Glick, S. M., Yalow, R. S. and Berson, S. A. (1963). Secretion of human growth hormone: physiologic and experimental modification. *Metabolism*, **12**, 577.
6 Danforth, E. and Rosenfeld, P. S. (1970). Effect of intravenous glucagon on circulating levels of growth hormone and 17-hydroxicorticosteroids. *J. Clin. Endocrinol. Metab.*, **30**, 117.
7 Milner, R. D. G. and Wright, A. D. (1966). Blood glucose, plasma insulin and growth hormone response to hyperglycaemia in the newborn. *Clin. Sci.*, **31**, 309.
8 Mitchell, M. L., Byrne, M. J. and Sawin, C. T. (1969). Growth hormone release by glucagon. *Lancet*, **i**, 289.
9 Podolsky, S. and Sivaprassad, R. (1972). Assessment of growth hormone reserve: comparison of intravenous arginine and subcutaneous glucagon stimulation tests. *J. Clin. Endocrinol. Metab.*, **35**, 580.
10 Mitchell, M. L., Byrne, M. J., Sanchez, Y. and Sawin, C. T. (1970). Detection of growth hormone deficiency. *N. Engl. J. Med.*, **282**, 539.
11 Cain, J. P., Williams, G. H. and Dluhy, R. G. (1970). Glucagon stimulation of human growth hormone. *J. Clin. Endocrinol. Metab.*, **31**, 222.
12 Mitchell, M. L., Suvunrungsi, P. and Sawin, C. (1971). Effect of propranolol on the response of serum growth hormone to glucagon. *J. Clin. Endocrinol. Metab.*; **32**, 470.

13 Wieland, R. G., Hallberg, M. C. and Zorn, E. M. (1973). Growth hormone response to intramuscular glucagon. *J. Clin. Endocrinol. Metab.*, **37,** 329.

14 Lefèbvre, P. J., Cession-Fossion, A., and Luyckv, A. S. (1966). Glucagon test for phaeochromocytoma. *Lancet,* **ii,** 1366.

15 Joasoo, A. and Freeman, A. (1967). Tyramine and glucagon in phaeochromocytoma. *Lancet,* **ii,** 726.

16 Lawrence, A. M. (1967). Glucagon provocative test for phaeochromocytoma. *Ann. Intern. Med.,* **66,** 1091.

17 Sheps, S. G. and Maher, F. T. (1968). Histamine and glucagon test in diagnosis of phaeochromocytoma. *J. Am. Med. Assoc.,* **205,** 895.

18 Brunner, H., Grabner, G., Michalek, G.P. and Paumgartner, G. (1968). Die Beurteilung der Leberfunktion mit Hilfe des Glukagon-Tests. *Wien. Z. Inn. Med.,* **49,** 409.

19 Grabner, G. and Neumayr, A. (1964). Probleme über Wechselbeziehungen zwischen Leberdurchblutung und Stoffwechsel. *Wien. Z. Inn. Med.,* **45,** 523.

20 Hardman, J. G., Davies, J. W. and Sutherland, E. W. (1969). Effects of some hormonal and other factors on the excretion of guanosine 3', 5'-monophosphate and adenosine 3', 5'-monophosphate in rat urine. *J. Biol. Chem.,* **244,** 6354.

21 Broadus, A. E., Kaminsky, N. I. and Northcutt, R. C. (1970). Effects of glucagon on adenosine 3', 5'-monophosphate in human plasma and urine. *J. Clin. Invest.,* **49,** 2237.

22 Strange, R. C. and Mjos, O. D. (1975). The sources of plasma cyclic AMP: studies in the rat using isoprenaline, nicotinic acid, and glucagon. *Eur. J. Clin. Invest.,* **5,** 147.

23 Davies, T. F., Prudhoe, K. and Douglas, A. P. (1976). Plasma cyclic adenosine 3', 5'-monophosphate response to glucagon in patients with liver disease. *Br. Med. J.,* **1,** 931.

24 Quirarte, C., Woodward, E. R. and Dragstedt, L. R. (1966). Glucagon and inhibition of gastric secretion. *Arch. Surg.,* **93,** 475.

25 Lin, T. M., Evans, D. C. and Spray, G. F. (1973). Mechanism studies of gastric inhibition by glucagon. Failure of KCl and adrenergic blocking agents to prevent its action. *Arch. Int. Pharmacodyn.,* **202,** 314.

26 Hess, A. F. (1913). The gastric secretion of infants at birth. *Ann. J. Dis. Child.,* **6,** 264.

27 Rogers, I. M., Davidson, D. C., Lawrence, J., Ardill, J. and Buchanan, K. D. (1974). Neonatal secretion of gastrin and glucagon. *Arch. Dis. Child.,* **49,** 796.

28 Konturek, S. J., Biernat, J., Kwiecen, N. and Olesky, J. (1975). Effect of glucagon on meal-induced gastric secretion in man. *Gastroenterology,* **68,** 448.

29 Gomez Pan, A., Reed, J. D., Albinus, M., Shaw, B., Hall, R., Besser, G. M., Coy, D. H., Kastin, A. J. and Schally, A. V. (1975). Direct inhibition of gastric acid and pepsin secretion by growth hormone release-inhibiting hormone in cats. *Lancet,* **i,** 888.

30 Albinus, M., Blair, E. L., Case, R. M., Coy, D. H., Gomez Pan, A., Hirst, B. H., Reed, J. D., Schally, A. V., Shaw, B., Smith, P. A. and Smy, J. R. (1977). Comparison of the effect of somatostatin on gastrointestinal function in the conscious and anaesthetized cat and on the isolated cat pancreas. *J. Physiol.*, **269,** 77.

31 Patton, G. S., Dobbs, R., Orci, L., Vale, W. and Unger, R. H. (1976). Stimulation of pancreatic immunoreactive somatostatin (IRS) release by glucagon. *Metabolism,* **25,** suppl. 1, 1499.

32 Parmley, W. M., Glick, G., and Sonnenblick, E. H. (1968). Cardiovascular effects of glucagon in man. *N. Engl. J. Med.,* **279,** 12.

33 Steiner, C., Wit, A. L. and Damato, A. N. (1976). Effects of glucagon on atrioventricular conduction and ventricular automaticity in dogs. *Circ. Res.,* **24,** 167.

34 Fazah, A. and Tuttle, R. (1960). Studies on the pharmacology of glucagon. *J. Pharmacol. Exp. Ther.,* **129,** 49.

35 Regan, T. J., Lehan, P. H., Henneman, D. H., Behar, A. and Hellems, H. K. (1964). Myocardial metabolic and contractile response to glucagon and epinephrine. *J. Lab. Clin. Med.,* **63,** 638.

36 Whitehouse, F. W. and James, T. N. (1966). Chronotropic action of glucagon on the sinus node. *Proc. Soc. Exp. Biol. Med.,* **122,** 823.

37 Brogan, E., Kozonis, M. C. and Overy, D. C. (1969). Glucagon therapy in heart failure. *Lancet,* **i,** 482.

38 Eddy, J. D., O'Brien, E. T. and Singh, S. P. (1969). Glucagon and haemodynamics of acute myocardial infarction. *Br. Med. J.,* **4,** 663.

39 Greenberg, B. H., Tsakiris, A. G. and Moffitt, E. A. (1970). The haemodynamic and metabolic effects of glucagon in patients with chronic valvular heart disease. *Mayo Clin. Proc.,* **45,** 132.

40 Murtagh, J. G., Binnion, P. F. and Lal, S. (1970). Haemodynamic effects of glucagon. *Br. Heart J.,* **32,** 307.

41 Nord, H. J., Fontanes, A. L. and Williams, J. F. (1970). Treatment of congestive heart failure with glucagon. *Ann. Intern Med.,* **72,** 649.

42 Wilcken, D. E. L. and Lvoff, R. (1970). Glucagon in resistant heart failure and cardiogenic shock. *Lancet,* **i,** 1315.

43 Fajans, S. S. (1976). Fasting hypoglycaemia in adults. *N. Engl. J. Med.,* **294,** 766.

44 Marks, V. (1971). Diagnosis of insulinoma. *Gut,* **12,** 835.

45 Khurana, R. C. and Nolan, S. (1971). Insulin and glucose patterns in control subjects and in proven insulinoma. *Am. J. Med. Sci.,* **262,** 115.

46 Marks, V. and Alberti, K. G. (1976). Selected tests of carbohydrate metabolism. *Clin. Endocrinol. Metab.,* **5,** 805.

2 The Physiological Role of Glucagon in the Gastro-intestinal Tract

D. L. Wingate and E. Pearce

INTRODUCTION

Since Stunkard et al.[1] showed that glucagon abolished gastric 'hunger contractions', there has been continuing interest in the possible role of pancreatic glucagon in the gastrointestinal tract. Clinically, the focus of attention has been centred on the abolition of intestinal motility demonstrated by Dotevall and Kock,[2] but numerous other studies have been performed. These studies are summarized in Tables 2.1 and 2.2, where an attempt has been made to express the concentrations of glucagon used in comparable terms, rather than invariably in the published dosage. The studies summarized in Table 2.1[1-32] cover aspects of gastrointestinal motility, absorption and blood flow, while those in Table 2.2[33-37] refer to studies on the lower oesophageal sphincter. There seems to be general agreement (Table 2.1) that glucagon is a splanchnic vasodilator, although the physiological importance of this effect is not clear; a recent study[8] emphasizes that the route of administration of glucagon may be of crucial importance. There is also reasonable agreement[33-37] that glucagon inhibits gastrin (or pentagastrin) stimulation of the lower oesophageal sphincter, but again there must be some doubt as to whether this is physiological, since Henderson and his colleagues[38] have suggested that the action of gastrin on the oesophageal sphincter is probably pharmacological rather than physiological.

The role, if any, of glucagon in the control of motility is less clear. Not only have some studies shown opposite effects,[29 32] but there are problems in the design and interpretation of such studies which have been discussed by Whalen[3]. Certainly

TABLE 2.1

Study	Target	Dose	Effect
(a) Isolated tissue			
Cameron et al. (1970)[3]	Human antrum	1 μg/ml	Nil
Gerner and Haffner (1975)[4]	Guinea-pig stomach	10 μg/ml (?)	Inhibition of pressure on distention only
Kowalewski et al. (1976)[5]	Perfused pig stomach	166 μg/min i.a.	Inhibition of electrical activity
(b) Animals: intra-arterial dosage			
Danford (1971)[6]	Dog	2.5 μg/kg	Abolition of digoxin-induced vaso-constriction in superior mesenteric artery
Fasth and Hultén (1971)[7]	(i) Cat	10–100 μg/kg/min (infusion)	Splanchnic vasodilatation decreased gut motility
	(ii) Adrenalectomized cat		Splanchnic vasodilatation normal motility
MacFerran and Mailman (1977)[8]	Dog	0.05 and 0.5 μg/kg/min	Increased intestinal splanchnic flow and fluid absorption

(c) Animals: single dose studies

Author	Animal	Dose	Effect
Hubel (1972)[9]	Rat	4–256 μg/kg i.v.	Increased fluid absorption
Johanssen and Segerström (1972)[10]	Rat	1.2–9.6 mg/kg s.c.	Retardation of gastric emptying
Kock et al. (1970)[11]	Dog	10 μg/kg i.v.	Reverses sympathetic effect on splanchnic bed
Lin et al. (1973)[12]	Dog	50 μg/kg	Inhibits gastric H^+ secretion
Necheles et al. (1966)[13]	Dog	6–313 μg/kg i.v.	Inhibits gastric and duodenal motility but not consistently
Stickney et al. (1958)[14]	Rat	7–280 μg/kg i.p.	No effect on motility
Tibblin (1970)[15]	Dog	10 μg/kg i.v.	Increased sup. mesenteric arterial flow
Višňovský (1976)[16]	Rat	2 mg/kg s.c.	Decreased gastric emptying and intestinal transit

(d) Animals: i.v. infusion studies

Author	Animal	Dose	Effect
Barbezat and Grossman (1971)[17]	Dog	0.5 μg/kg/min	Increased intestinal secretion
Krarup and Larsen (1974)[18]	Cat	0.1–5 μg/kg/min	Reverses sympathetic effect on splanchnic bed

Superior figures denote references at end of Chapter.

TABLE 2.1 continued

Study	Target	Dose	Effect
Rudo and Rosenberg (1972)[19]	Rat	(Chronic intra-peritoneal injection: 0.3 μg/kg 6-hourly for 6 days).	Increased intestinal sugar transport
Scott and Summers (1976)[20]	Rat	1, 10, 100 μg/kg/min	Inhibition of jejunal contraction and transit of higher dose levels
Tibblin (1970)[15]	Dog	0.1 μg/kg/min	Increased sup. mesenteric arterial flow
Valenzuela (1976)[21]	Dog	0.1–0.4 μg/kg/min	Decreased intragastric pressure
Wingate et al. (1977)[22]	Dog	0.04–0.32 μg/kg/min	Stimulation of intestinal myoelectric activity
(e) Man: single dose studies			
Dotevall and Kock (1963)[2]	Jejunum and colon	3.6–14.3 μg/kg i.v.	Inhibition of motility for 10 min
Kock et al. (1967)[23]	Jejunum and colon	0.7–1.4 μg/kg i.p. and i.v.	Inhibition of motility for 4–8 min
Ratzman and Knoke (1974)[24]	Stomach	14 μg/kg	Inhibition of basal H$^+$ secretion

22

Reference	Region	Dose	Effect
Stoddard and Duthie (1976)[25]	Stomach	5–10 μg/kg	Biphasic effect on B.E.R.
Stunkard et al. (1955)[1]	Stomach	28 μg/kg	Inhibition of hunger contractions
(f) Man: infusion studies			
Chowdhury et al. (1976)[26]	Rectosigmoid in constipation	0.17 μg/kg/min	Similar effect to atropine on hyperactive segment
Chowdhury and Larber (1977)[27]	Distal colon and rectum	0.5 μg/kg/min	Inhibition of food or morphine-stimulated activity
Corazziara et al. (1973)[28]	Duodenum and jejunum	0.5–1.0 μg/kg/min	Abolition of movement: duodenal but *not* jejunal stasis
Hicks and Turnberg (1974)[29]	Jejunum	0.02 μg/kg/min	Increased rate of transit
Konturek et al. (1975)[30]	Stomach	0.09–0.7 μg/kg/min	Inhibition of food-stimulated H^+ secretion
Paul (1974)[31]	Stomach and colon	0.1 μg/kg/min	Inhibition of motility
Stunkard et al. (1955)[1]	Stomach	0.6 μg/kg/min	Inhibition of 'hunger contraction'
Whalen et al. (1973)[32]	Small intestine	Arginine infusion	Prolongation of transit with rise in plasma glucagon (81 to 214 pg/ml)

Superior figures denote references at end of chapter.

TABLE 2.2

Study	Species	Dose	Route	Effect
Hogan et al. (1975)[33]	Man	0.014–1.4 µg/kg	Rapid i.v.	Inhibition of pentagastrin-stimulated pressure at low doses, resting pressure at higher doses
Jaffer et al. (1974)[34]	Man	10 µg/kg Arginine	Rapid i.v. i.v. infusion	Inhibition of resting and stimulated pressure No effect
Jennewein et al. (1973)[35]	{ Man Dog	60 µg/kg 100 µg/kg	Rapid i.v. Rapid i.v.	Inhibition Inhibition and pentagastrin antagonism
Waldeck et al. (1973)[36]	Man	1–100 µg/kg	Rapid i.v.	Inhibition of resting and stimulated pressure, maximal at 30 µg/kg
Wu et al. (1975)[37]	Z–E pts.	0.014–0.14 µg/kg	Rapid i.v.	Fall of resting pressure

Superior figures denote references at end of chapter.

dosage is important; one study[40] has been omitted from Table 2.1 as the dosage of glucagon employed was not stated. More than that, it is not always possible to deduce the effect of a substance on the intestinal smooth muscle from pressure or transit studies; moreover pressure changes do not define transit changes, and *vice versa*.

Surprisingly, there has been almost no interest in the effect of glucagon on myoelectric activity, although myoelectric activity is a reliable index of contractile activity. One study in the isolated vascular-perfused stomach,[5] using a large dose, demonstrated inhibition of electrical activity, but the effects on intestinal myoelectric activity are not known.

Recently, there have been suggestions[7][41] that the apparent inhibition of motility by glucagon may be a secondary effect due to glucagon-stimulated adrenergic inhibition. At the same time, the last decade has seen a new understanding of gastrointestinal myoelectric activity with the description of physiological patterns of activity.[42] There has also been increasing interest in the possible control of such activity by gastrointestinal peptides, and insulin has been postulated as playing an important role.[43] Meanwhile, the discovery of large numbers of cells in the digestive mucosa containing 'enteroglucagon', a peptide with immunological affinities with pancreatic glucagon,[44] has indicated the need for further study.

We have studied the effects of pancreatic glucagon on canine intestinal myoelectric activity using a technique[45] which allows quantitation of the incidence of spike activity. Until enteroglucagon is available for study, the use of pancreatic glucagon as a structural analogue – and a possible functional analogue – seems reasonable. The administration of the peptide by slow infusion, rather than as a 'bolus', was chosen to give an experimental protocol which was uniform with similar studies on other gastrointestinal peptides.[46]

METHODS

The subjects were 6 retriever dogs (weight 25–27 kg) who had electrodes implanted on the serosal surface of the distal duodenum, mid-jejunum and terminal ileum, under aseptic surgery up to 6 months earlier. Before surgery, the dogs had been trained to rest quietly supported by a sling over prolonged periods. During the 6 hours of each study, the dogs were alert, responsive, and showed no signs of distress.

Before each study, the dogs were fasted for 18 hours and two venous cannulae were inserted for infusion and sampling respectively. Each study comprised three consecutive 2-hour periods, and physiological saline was infused throughout at 24 ml per hour. Glucagon (Novo Laboratories Ltd.) was added to the saline infusion for the middle 2 hours of each study to give 0.5, 0.25, 0.125 or 0.06 mg/h. (equivalent to 0.32, 0.16, 0.08 and 0.04 μg/kg/min) or administered as a rapid intravenous injection of 1 mg (40 μg/kg) in 2 minutes at the end of the first 2-hour period. 5 ml samples of blood were withdrawn at the start, and then 60, 120, 125, 130, 135, 150, 165, 180, 195, 210, 240, 300 and 360 minutes later. During the 6 hours, myoelectric activity from the three electrode sites was recorded continuously on C120 $\frac{1}{8}''$ magnetic tape cassettes (Phillips) using a Medilog 4-24 cassette tape recorder (Oxford Electronic Instruments, Abingdon, Oxon.).

The recorded myoelectric activity was analysed during rapid replay;[46] this analysis yielded numerical counts of spike activity at each site for each 2-hour period, and also a graphic histogram of spikes per minute at each site for the whole study. Glucose was assayed in all blood samples within 15 minutes of sampling using a rapid quantitative glucose oxidase method ('Glucoscan', Portex Ltd., Hythe, Kent). After separation, serum samples were stored at -18 °C for subsequent radio-immunoassay for insulin.[47]

RESULTS

The infusion of 1 mg of glucagon in two hours resulted in a statistically significant increase in the incidence of spike activity (Figure 2.1). This was most marked in the jejunum, where the number of spikes was approximately trebled. This overall increase in spike activity was accompanied by abolition of the fasting pattern of cyclical migrating complexes (Figure 2.2) to a

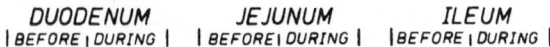

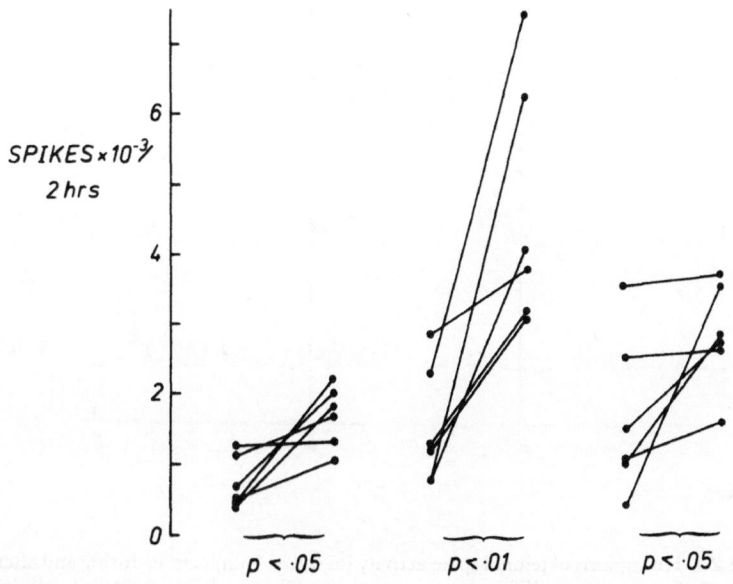

Figure 2.1 Comparison of total spike activity at three levels of the intestine in 6 dogs for 2 hours before and 2 hours during infusion of glucagon (0.5 mg/h) ·

pattern resembling that seen after food. The fasting pattern was abolished at all three levels of the small intestine, and the duration of the pattern change extended throughout the infusion period; at the end of the infusion period there was an abrupt reversion to the normal fasting pattern (Figure 2.2).

Lower infusion doses of glucagon produced a similar enhancement of spike activity, and abolition of fasting patterns (Figure 2.2). At a dose of 0.125 mg/h there is clear disruption of the fasting pattern; no periods of absent spike activity are seen during the peptide infusion, but they are seen preceding and following the glucagon infusion. At the lowest dose (0.06 mg/h), the effect is equivocal; a perturbation of spike activity is seen, but the record also suggests the persistence of cyclic change (Figure 2.2).

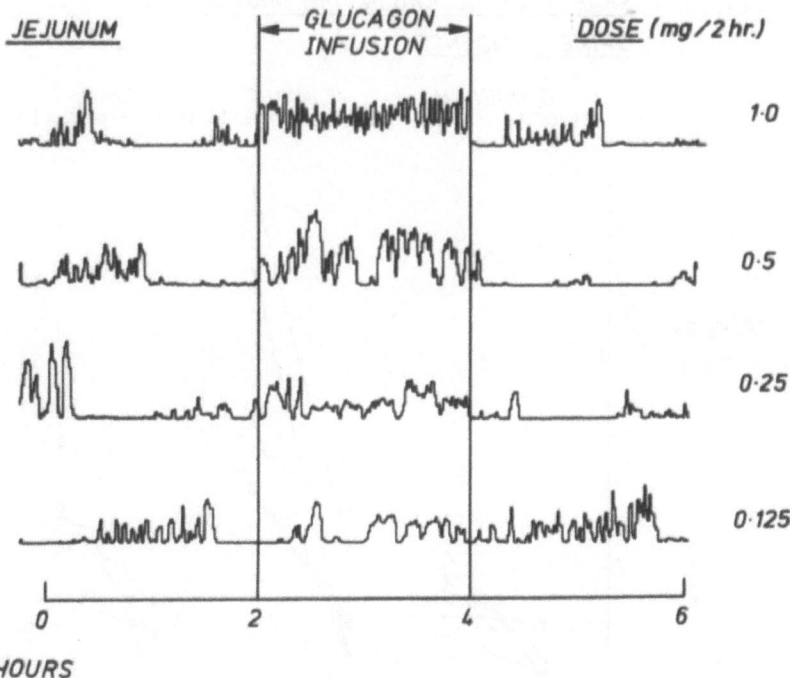

Figure 2.2 Histograms of jejunal spike activity (as spikes/min) before, during and after glucagon infusion at four different concentrations. All records show cyclical activity before and after glucagon

Glucagon administered by rapid injection inhibits spike activity, as shown in Figure 2.3. In the study illustrated, the injection was given just after the passage of a migrating myoelectric complex (MMC) in the duodenum, and just before the peak of the same complex in the jejunum. The effect of the injection was the extreme attenuation of the next duodenal MMC, about one hour after the injection, and the attenuation of the peak of the jejunal MMC just after the injection.

The insulin and glucose response to 1 mg of glucagon as either a rapid injection or a 2-hour infusion is illustrated in Figure 2.4. The effect of injection is an immediate and sustained hyperglycaemia, with only a moderate and brief rise in insulin. By contrast, infusion has a more marked effect on insulin, while the rise in blood sugar is smaller. The peak insulin concentrations during infusion are within the range of insulin response

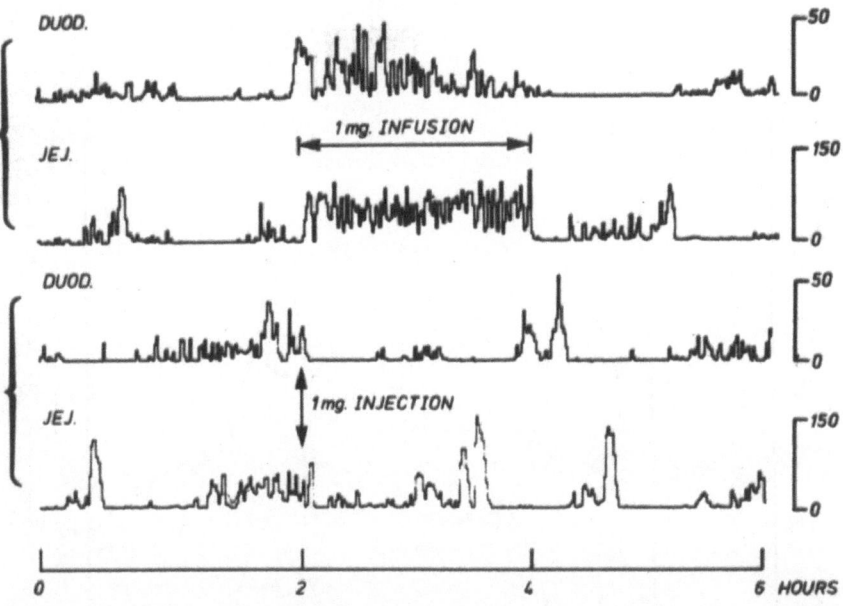

Figure 2.3 Histograms of duodenal and jejunal spike activity showing the response to infusion of 1 mg glucagon in 2 hours (upper 2 records) and to rapid injection of 1 mg glucagon (lower 2 records)

that we have observed in the same animals in response to a normal meal, using the same assay.[48]

DISCUSSION

These findings show that the effect of glucagon on intestinal motor activity is stimulation, and not inhibition, when it is administered as a constant infusion. Moreover, the stimulatory effect of the peptide is evident even when the infusion dose is lowered.

These results prompt several questions. First, how do these studies on myoelectric activity relate to 'motility'? Studies such as these are not possible in man. Nevertheless, there is good evidence that spikes are the electrical correlate of contractile activity.[49] The absence of spikes after glucagon injection (Figure 2.3) represents a non-motile intestine, and this is consistent with the motility inhibition found in other studies.[1 2 23] Equally, the intense but irregular spike activity seen on

29

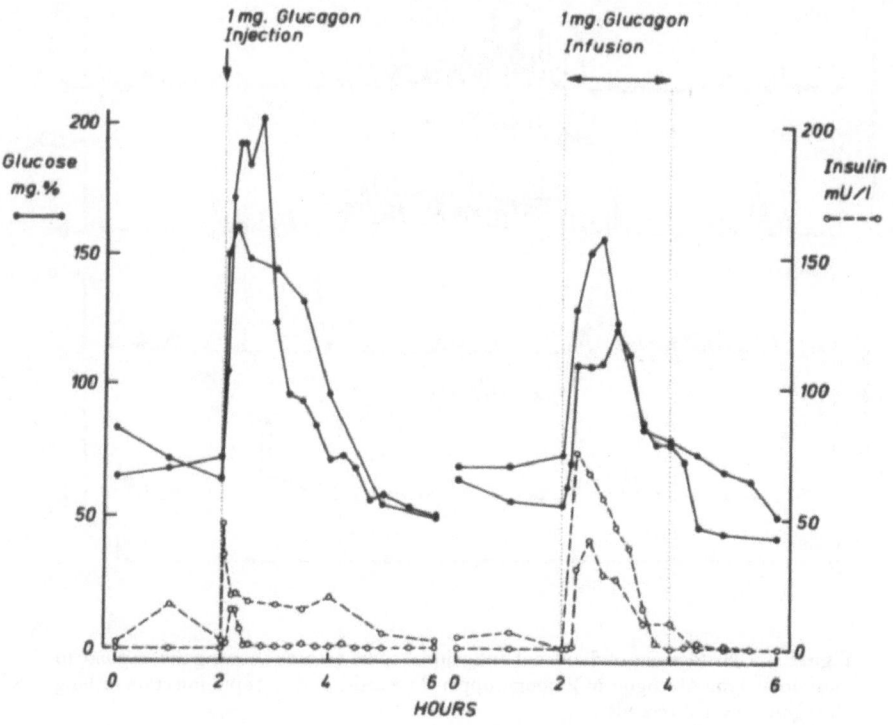

Figure 2.4 Comparison of changes in plasma insulin (open circles) and glucose (closed circles) in 2 studies of glucagon infusion (right) and 2 studies of glucagon injection (left), as illustrated in Figure 2.3

glucagon infusion represents contractile activity of the type seen after feeding – segmentation with slow propulsion. In this respect, our studies are consistent with the observations of Whalen *et al.*,[32] who demonstrated delayed transit.

Secondly, are these studies relevant to man? The cyclical fasting activity first found in dogs[42] has been demonstrated in other mammalian species, and more recently in man using pressure recording techniques.[50] Certainly the inhibitory effect of rapid glucagon injection in man[2] has been reproduced here in the dog, and it seems reasonable to speculate that the converse effect of glucagon infusion will have similar effects in man.

Thirdly, how is glucagon acting? It seems likely that the effect of a glucagon bolus is adrenergic stimulation,[7] and possibly also a vagal effect.[41] Our studies show prolongation of the inhibitory effect (Figure 2.3 and 2.4) long after the exogenous peptide must have disappeared, and this is consistent with an indirect action. The stimulatory effect of glucagon may be a direct effect, since the duration of stimulation (Figure 2.2 and 2.3) coincides precisely with the duration of the infusion. It has been claimed that insulin may disrupt the fasting pattern,[43] but the data shown in Figure 2.4 do not support the hypothesis that the motor stimulation is due to either hyperglycaemia or hyperinsulinaemia, since both were abolished *before* the end of the infusion; again this is consistent with the studies of Whalen *et al.*[32] On the basis of the present data, a direct effect of glucagon on the intestine seems most likely.

Finally are these results 'physiological' and do they explain the function of enteroglucagon? Certainly our dosage was low in comparison with other studies (Table 2.1 (d)), but even the lowest dose of infusion used by us is 'unphysiological' in that it exceeds the dose of glucagon required to simulate postprandial plasma levels (S. R. Bloom, personal communication). All that can be claimed is that it is perhaps more physiological and less pharmacological than the rapid injection of a large dose. If – and it has yet to be proved – studies on pancreatic glucagon bear any relation to enteroglucagon, our findings make more physiological sense.

Of the peptides that we have tested using this study protocol (motilin,[51] pentagastrin,[46] cholecystokinin[46] and secretin[46]), glucagon is the only one which has produced a pattern closely resembling the pattern of motor activity induced by food.[48] Since the known effect of food is to produce irregular but persistent spiking activity, whose motor correlate is segmentation rather than rapid propulsion, it has been difficult to assign a significant role to a peptide previously assumed to inhibit motor activity. When Bloom[52] stated that 'it seems reasonable to hypothesise that enteroglucagon acts to inhibit motility when absorbed food passed down the gut', the myoelectric correlates of feeding were as yet unknown, but our observations add some weight to his speculation. Enteric glucagon remains an unknown functional entity, but our findings suggest that it may prove to be an important mediator of the motor response to food. This would be consistent with what must be regarded as the only gastrointestinal physiological property of glucagon on which there is reasonable agreement: vasodilation and increased flow in the splanchnic bed, which is another response to feeding.

Acknowledgements

Financial support from the Wellcome Trust and the Medical Research Council, and technical and bibliographic assistance from Novo Laboratories Ltd., is gratefully acknowledged. Anne Ling and Michael Hutton worked with Elizabeth Pearce on the experimental work described in this paper, and it is to them that the credit is due. Dr B. J. Boucher kindly carried out the radioimmunoassay, and Dr P. J. Warren provided a 'Glucoscan'. Thanks are also due to Dr David Morris, for helpful advice on the design of this work.

References

1 Stunkard, A. J., van Itallie, T. B. and Reis, B. B. (1955). The mechanism of satiety: Effect of glucagon on gastric hunger contractions in man. *Proc. Soc. Exp. Biol.*, **89,** 258.

2 Dotevall, G. and Kock, N. G. (1963). Effect of glucagon on intestinal motility in man. *Gastroenterology*, **45,** 364.

3 Cameron, A. J., Phillips, S. F. and Summerskill, W. H. J. (1970). Comparison of effects of gastrin, cholecystokinin–pancreozymin, secretin, and glucagon on human stomach muscle in vitro. *Gastroenterology*, **59,** 539.

4 Gerner, T. and Haffner, J. F. W. (1975). X – The significance of distention for the effect of glucagon on the fundic and antral motility in isolated guinea pig stomach. *Scand. J. Gastroenterol.*, **10** (suppl. 35), 51.

5 Kowalewski, K., O'Sullivan, G. and Kokodej, A. (1976). Effect of glucagon on myoelectrical and mechanical activity of the isolated homologous perfused porcine stomach. *Pharmacology*, **14,** 115.

6 Danford, R. O. (1971). The splanchnic vasoconstrictive effect of digoxin and its reversal by glucagon. In J. Scott, (ed.), *Vascular Disorders of the Intestine*, p. 421. (New York: Boley).

7 Fasth, S. and Hultén, L. (1971). The effect of glucagon on intestinal motility and blood flow. *Acta Physiol. Scand.*, **83,** 169.

8 MacFerran, S. N. and Mailman, D. (1977). Effects of glucagon on canine intestinal sodium and water fluxes and regional blood flow. *J. Physiol.*, **266,** 1.

9   Hubel, K. A. (1972). Effects of secretin and glucagon on intestinal transport of ions and water in rat. *Proc. Exp. Biol. Med.,* **139,** 656.

10 Johansson, H. and Segerström, A. (1972). Glucagon and gastrointestinal motility in relation to thyroid–parathyroid function. *Upsals. J. Med. Sci.,* **77,** 183.

11 Kock, N. G., Tibblin, S. and Schenk, W. G. (1971). Modification by glucagon on the splanchnic vascular responses to activation of the sympathicoadrenal system. *J. Surg. Res.,* **1,** 12.

12 Lin, T. M., Evans, D. C. and Spray, G. F. (1973). Mechanism studies of gastric inhibition by glucagon: Failure of KCl and adrenergic blocking agents to prevent its action. *Arch. Int. Pharmacodyn.,* **202,** 314.

13 Necheles, H., Sporn, J. and Walker, L. (1966). Effect of glucagon on gastrointestinal motility. *Am. J. Gastroenterol.,* **45,** 34.

14 Stickney, J. C., Northup, D. W. and van Liere, E. J. (1958). Effect of glucagon on propulsive motility of rat small intestine. *Fed. Proc.,* **17,** 157.

15 Tibblin, S. (1970). Splanchnic hemodynamic responses to glucagon. *Arch. Surg.,* **100,** 84.

16 Visnovský, P. (1976). Effect of corticosterone, glucagon and growth hormone on gastrointestinal propulsive motility in rats. *Bratisl. Lek. Listy,* **65,** 394.

17 Barbezat, G. and Grossman, M. (1971). Effect of glucagon on water and electrolyte movement in jejunum and ileum of dog. *Gastroenterology,* **60,** 762.

18 Krarup, N. and Larsen, J. A. (1974). The effect of glucagon on hepatosplanchnic hemodynamics, functional capacity, and metabolism of the liver in cats. *Acta Physiol. Scand.,* **91,** 42.

19 Rudo, N. D. and Rosenberg, I. H. (1972). Chronic glucagon administration enhances intestinal transport in the rat. *Fed. Proc.,* No. 166.

20 Scott, L. D. and Summers, R. W. (1976). Correlation of contractions and transit in rat small intestine. *Am. J. Physiol.,* **230,** 132.

21 Valenzuela, J. E. (1976). Effect of intestinal hormones and peptides on intragastric pressure in dogs. *Gastroenterology,* **71,** 766.

22 Wingate, D. L., Morris, D. and Thomas, P. A. (1977). Glucagon stimulates intestinal motor activity. *Gut,* **18,** A966.

23 Kock, N.G., Darle, N. and Dotevall, G. (1967). Inhibition of intestinal motility in man by glucagon given intraportally. *Gastroenterology,* **53,** 88.

24 Ratzmann, K. P. and Knoke, M. (1974). Glukagon und seine Wirkung auf den Gastrointestinaltrakt. *Zschr. Inn. Med.,* **29,** 94.

25 Stoddard, C. J. and Duthie, H.L. (1976). Effect of vagotomy on the response of gastric myoelectrical activity to glucagon and food. *Scand. J. Gastroenterol.,* **11** (suppl. 42), 77.

26 Chowdhury, A. R., Dinoso, V. P. and Lorber, S. H. (1976). Characterization of a hyperactive segment at the rectosigmoid junction. *Gastroenterology,* **71,** 584.

27 Chowdhury, A. R. and Lorber, S. H. (1977). Effects of glucagon and secretin on food- or morphine-induced motor activity of the distal colon, rectum, and anal sphincter. *Digest Dis.,* **22,** 775.

28   Corazziari, E., Habib, I. F., Delle Fave, G. and Torsoli, A. (1973). Effets de certaines hormones gastro-intestinales sur la motricité duodéno-jéjunale. *Biol. Gastro-Enterol.*, **6,** 368.

29   Hicks, T. and Turnberg, L. A. (1974). Influence of glucagon on the human jejunum. *Gastroenterology*, **67,** 1114.

30   Konturek, S. J., Biernat, J., Kwiecien, N. and Oleksy, J. (1975). Effect of glucagon on meal-induced gastric secretion in man. *Gastroenterology*, **68,** 448.

31   Paul, F. (1974). Quantitative Untersuchungen der Wirkung von Pankreasglukagon und Sekretin auf die Magen-Darm-Motorik Mittels elektromanometrischen Simultanregistrierungen beim Menschen. *Klin. Wochenschr.*, **52,** 983.

32   Whalen, G. E., Wu, W. C., Ganeshappa, K. P., Wall, M. J., Kalkhoff, R. K. and Soergel, K. H. (1973). The effect of endogenous glucagon on human small bowel function. *Gastroenterology*, **64,** 822.

33   Hogan, W. J., Dodds, W. J., Hoke, S. E., Reid, D. P., Kalkhoff, R. K. and Arndorfer, R. C. (1975). Effect of glucagon on esophageal motor function. *Gastroenterology*, **69,** 160.

34   Jaffer, S. S., Makhlouf, G. M., Schorr, B. A., and Zfass, A. M. (1974). Nature and kinetics of inhibition of lower esophageal sphincter pressure by glucagon. *Gastroenterology*, **67,** 42.

35   Jennewein, H. M., Waldeck, F., Siewert, R., Weiser, F. and Thimm, R. (1973). The interaction of glucagon and pentagastrin on the lower oesophageal sphincter in man and dog. *Gut*, **14,** 861.

36   Waldeck, F., Siewert, R., Jennewein, H. M. and Weiser, F. (1973). Das Druckprofil im unteren Osophagussphinkter beim Menschen und seine Beeinflussung durch Gastrin, Calcitonin und Glukagon. *Dtsch. Med. Wschr.*, **98,** 1059.

37   Wu, W. C., Hogan, W. J., Whalen, G. E., Hoke, S. E., Go, V. L. W. and Kalkoff, R. K. (1975). Lower esophageal sphincter responses to enteric hormones in two patients with Zollinger–Ellison syndrome. *Digest Dis.*, **20,** 716.

38   Henderson, J. M., Lidgard, G., Osborne, D. H., Carter, D. C. and Heading, R. C. (1978). Lower oesophageal sphincter response to gastrin - pharmacological or physiological? *Gut*, **19,** 99.

39   Whalen, G. E. (1974). Glucagon and the small gut. *Gastroenterology*, **67,** 1284.

40   Sporn, J. and Necheles, H. (1956). Effect of glucagon on gastrointestinal motility. *Am. J. Physiol.*, **187,** 634.

41   Miolan, J. P. and Roman, C. (1975). Mechanisms of the inhibitory effect of glucagon on gastric motility. *Proc. 5th Int. Symp. Gastrointest. Motility*, p. 70. (Herentals: Typoff Press).

42   Szurszewski, J. H. (1969). A migrating complex of the canine small intestine. *Am. J. Physiol.*, **217,** 1757.

43   Bueno, L. and Ruckebusch, M. (1976). Insulin and jejunal electrical activity in dogs and sheep. *Am. J. Physiol.*, **230,** 1528.

44   Polak, J. M., Bloom, S. R., Coulling, I. and Pearse, A. G. E. (1971). Immuno-fluorescent localization of enteroglucagon in the gastrointestinal tract of the dog. *Gut*, **12**, 311.

45   Wingate, D. L., Barnett, T. G., Green, W. E. R. and Armstrong-James, M. (1977). Automated high-speed analysis of gastrointestinal myoelectric activity. *Am. J. Digest Dis.*, **22**, 243.

46   Wingate, D. L., Pearce, E. A., Hutton, M., Dand, A., Thompson, H. H. and Wunsch, E. (1978). Quantitative comparison of the effects of cholecystokinin, secretin, and pentagastrin on gastrointestinal myoelectric activity in the conscious fasted dog. *Gut*, **19**, 593.

47   Morgan, C. R. and Lazarow, A. (1963). Immunoassay of insulin: two antibody systems. *Diabetes*, **12**, 115.

48   Wingate, D. L., Thompson, H. H., Pearce, E. A., and Dand, A. (1977). Quantitative analysis of the effect of feeding canine intestinal myoelectric activity. *Gastroenterology*, **72**, A-128/1151.

49   Grivel, M. L. and Ruckebusch, Y. (1972). The propagation of segmental contractions along the small intestine. *J. Physiol.*, **227**, 611.

50   Vantrappen, G., Janssen, J., Hellemans, J. and Ghoos, Y. (1977). The interdigestive motor complex of normal subjects and patients with bacterial overgrowth of the small intestine. *J. Clin. Invest.*, **59**, 1158.

51   Wingate, D. L., Ruppin, H., Thompson, H. H., Green, W. E. R., Domschke, W., Wunch, E., Demling, L. and Ritchie, H. D. (1977). The gastrointestinal myoelectric response to 13-Nle-motilin infusion during interdigestive and digestive states in the conscious dog. *Acta Hep. Gastroenterol.*, **24**, 278.

52   Bloom, S. R. (1974). Glucagon: pancreatic and enteric. In W. Y. Chey and F. P. Brooks (eds.), *Endocrinology of the Gut*, pp. 88–102. (Thorofare, New Jersey: Chas. B. Slack).

DISCUSSION

Myren: I get the impression that the effect shown is a dose-dependent one. The effects seen with a high dose are quite different from those seen with a low one. This may account for the differences between infusion and syringe injections. For a valid observation one should relate the effects seen to the concentrations of glucagon in the blood.

Wingate: We have not done this. We are doing some blood studies now, and it is the opinion of Dr Bloom of Hammersmith Hospital in London that our infusion dose is some five times greater than the dose needed to produce physiological elevations of glucose in the plasma.

This brings us to the specific question of exactly what is the correct dose of glucagon. It seems to me that much depends on the route of administration. The half-life of glucagon is about eight minutes, but there is also the problem of access to the target organ. Before one can say what the correct dose is, one must know exactly what motor effect one is trying to achieve.

Paul: Your findings are in contrast to the results of our motility measurements with small micro-balloons. We infused glucagon intravenously or injected it. We controlled the action of glucagon by measuring the blood sugar level – at that time we did not have the RIA – and in all our experiments the blood sugar rose when we gave 0.05 mg over thirty minutes for two hours. We found that the motility in the stomach, the duodenum, and the colon was inhibited in all subjects. Could it be that species differences account for the different findings?

Wingate: A little, phehaps.

Paul: You said that the spike activity is necessary in order to get pressure waves. When one cannot find pressure waves, then, one may presume that there is no spike activity. There must, therefore, be a correlation between these two phenomena.

Kreel: Before you answer that, I would like to say that if you look at the dosage from the radiologist's viewpoint it is extremely interesting. Roscoe Miller of Indianapolis in the USA has done a lot of work with intramuscular dosages of 1 mg and 2 mg glucagon. He relates activity to the calibre of small bowel, and he relates the blood levels of glucose to bowel calibre. It seems that barium will reach the terminal ileum more quickly with 1 mg than with 2 mg.

Wingate: To come back to Professor Paul's point, I would be surprised if there was a species difference of this magnitude. I know of a group at Nottingham University in England which has done studies in dogs in a way similar to ours with the same results. There may be a species difference – others have tried similar studies in the pig and not found the same thing, but there may have been technical complications here – but I think it is more a matter of which region of the gut one studies. I would not be surprised if there is one effect in the colon and another in the stomach, for instance. Our target organ here is the mid-small intestine. This is an area which could probably be studied radiologically, but this seems rarely to have been done. I think that new sorts of studies will probably be done in man in the next year or two, because new systems using transducers, catheters, and so on, have recently been made available.

Paul: When we studied the third part of the duodenum we also got different results from yours.

Wingate: Yes, but the stimulation of the duodenum is not very great. It is with an infusion, and in particular in the jejunum, that we get an enormous stimulation.

Jaspan: Have you ever seen the effect on catecholamines induced by infusion as opposed to injection?

Wingate: No, we have not, ourselves, looked at catecholamines. Our hypothesis is based on other people's work on catecholamine release, and on experiments on adrenalectomized cats.

Jaspan: It may be that an infusion depletes the catecholamines, whereas an injection actually causes an acute release, doesn't it?

Wingate: Yes, certainly.

Volpicelli: Would you be willing to speculate on what impact these studies might have with regard to digestion? It is very difficult to relate disturbances in motility to digestive abnormalities.

Wingate: Perhaps I may, very briefly, put into context what this kind of interdigestive cycling means in terms of digestive physiology or digestive function. We are, of course, normally very rarely in an interdigestive phase, but we believe that this can increase because of a failure to switch on the feeding pattern, or, if you like, to switch off the cycling activity. It may be that in certain abnormal conditions the cycling activity continues after food and it may be this that propels the bile acids into the colon in people who have had vagotomies, causing post-vagotomy diarrhoea. If glucagon can switch on the feeding pattern, or switch off the fasting pattern, this is important. If this is the case, a peptide which is safe, and which, in people in whom this would not otherwise happen, will mimic the effect of food, could be clinically valuable in inducing correct digestive activity.

To a large extent, of course, this is speculation based on very little data, but it is significant because if there is going to be a clinical syndrome associated with this area of physiological phenomena (and there probably is) it is going to centre around the failure to produce proper feeding activity.

We have tried glucagon in post-operative paralytic ileus in the dog and in one case – in only one, because it is very difficult to get a reproducible state of ileus in the dog – we found that during the glucagon infusion there was complete relief of ileus. This is an area which we are now studying, but it really is too early to be very certain of the clinical correlations.

Paul: I am interested in your observation that if you inject glucagon or infuse it for a couple of hours you find inhibition of pressure waves, and if you infuse it for days the patient never gets an ileus. We have infused glucagon for more than eight days, and have never observed an ileus. There seems to be no explanation for this phenomenon at the moment.

3 The Role of Glucagon in Different Endoscopic Procedures in the Upper Gastrointestinal Tract

J. Myren

Endoscopy of the upper gastrointestinal tract is performed more frequently than all other endoscopical procedures added together. Of 321 478 diagnostic procedures collected from 28 centres for the study of complications at the Sixth World Congress of Gastroenterology (Madrid, June 1978), 194 909 were performed in the upper gastrointestinal tract. Most of these dealt with the duodenum, stomach, or lower part of the oesophagus, and were carried out to investigate neoplasms, ulcers, or the cause of bleedings.

The detection of pathological changes is highly dependent on optimal conditions for the observation of details. For detection of minimal changes, secretion and motility should be suppressed as much as possible. On the other hand, for the study of infiltrating processes, observation of motility may be helpful. Good relaxation of motility and inhibition of secretory processes are also required for a satisfactory examination of the cause of bleedings, and for a successful cannulation of the papilla of Vater.

In recent years therapeutic procedures have been performed in an increasing number of cases. Of a total of 8937 such procedures collected for the above-mentioned study, 2109 were polypectomies of the stomach, 862 were papillotomies, and 226 were performed in order to stop bleedings. Success in such instances, and the prevention of complications, is largely dependent on a satisfactory premedication providing good relaxation with a minimum of secretion.

The incidence of complications, such as bleedings and perforations, depends partly on the skill of the operator, but

39

also, and to a large extent, on successful premedication. In the above-mentioned survey, bleedings and perforations occurred in one case per 4000 examinations, and death occurred at the rate of one in approximately 40000. The death rate in patients examined by means of endoscopic retrograde cholangio-pancreaticography is some 20 times higher (0.05%), and in those subjected to papillotomy, as high as 1.16%.

It has been observed in recent years that 1–2 mg glucagon given intravenously decreases the tone and contraction of the gastrointestinal tract when studied by roentgen examination.[1-3] It has also been shown that similar doses of glucagon decrease the motility and secretion of the stomach and pancreas. This drug has, therefore, been used in the treatment of acute pancreatitis, but, in spite of the inhibitory effect on the pancreatic secretion, so far no effect on mortality has been demonstrated. A double-blind study has also shown its beneficial effect in endoscopic retrograde cholangio-pancreaticography (ERCP),[4] and, because of its relaxing effect on the sphincter of Oddi, it has also been used in the treatment of patients with biliary calculi.[5-7]

The purpose of the present communication is to answer the following questions:

(a) Is glucagon a useful premedication for diagnostic purposes in the upper gastrointestinal tract?

(b) Is glucagon useful for therapeutic purposes in the upper gastrointestinal tract?

GLUCAGON AS PREMEDICATION FOR DIAGNOSTIC PURPOSES

Several studies have shown that single intravenous infusions of 0.5–1 mg glucagon have been used for peroral endoscopy of the upper gastrointestinal tract.[8-13] These investigations have suggested that glucagon is of benefit by decreasing tonicity and motility for 10–15 minutes, thus facilitating the endoscopic observations. Two of these studies are discussed below.

Study 1 (Melsom *et al.*[12])
The question asked in this study was: Is glucagon a better

premedication than the conventional one of 50 mg pethidine plus 0.5 mg atropine for upper gastrointestinal endoscopy?

The material consisted of 30 male patients aged 42–64 with an average age of 55. (Table 3.1.) None had previously been operated upon. After an overnight fast they were given 0.5 mg glucagon (Novo) or 50 mg pethidine plus 0.5 mg atropine intravenously.

TABLE 3.1 Comparison of glucagon and pethidine + atropine

Observations	Glucagon	Pethidine + atropine
No. of patients	15	15
Mean age (range)	55 (42–64)	56 (47–63)
Previous peroral endoscopy	4	2
Clinical diagnosis		
Duodenal ulcer	3	4
Gastric ulcer	5	2
Gastritis	5	4
Oesophagitis	0	1
No abnormality	2	4

The material was coded into one group receiving glucagon (group G) and one receiving pethidine plus atropine (group PA).[15]

The results showed that a highly significant difference was observed between G and PA concerning the degree of vomiting, subjective discomfort, and the amount of gastric secretion, all of which were less in the PA group. In this group the salivation was also less than in the G group (Table 3.2). In the G group a

**TABLE 3.2 Comparison of the effect of glucagon with that of
pethidine + atropine. Significances indicated by _p_ values**

Findings	Glucagon	Pethidine + atropine
Decrease in		
vomiting		0.001
discomfort		0.001
secretion		0.001
salivation		0.001
motility	0.038	
pyloric reflux		NS
pyloric contraction		NS
Success of examination		NS

NS = no significance

significant prolongation of the inhibition of the antral and
duodenal motility was found ($p = 0.038$). The examinations
were considered equally successful in both groups, and no
adverse reactions were observed.

The results of this study thus showed that glucagon
premedication inhibits motility in the antrum and duodenum
for a longer period of time than pethidine and atropine.

This observation indicates the usefulness of glucagon in
patients in whom sedation is not wanted but in whom a quiet
antrum and duodenum is essential for a successful result of endoscopical procedure.

Study 2 (Qvigstad et al.[13])
In this double-blind study the effect of glucagon was more

TABLE 3.3 Comparison of glucagon and atropine – mean age and range

Premedication	No. of patients	Female	Male	Mean age years	Age range
Glucagon	12	6	6	62	56–70
Atropine	12	6	6	62	57–71
Placebo	12	6	6	63	55–69

precisely compared with the effect of atropine. The question posed was: Is glucagon a better premedication for upper gastrointestinal endoscopy than atropine alone?

This study involved 36 patients, 18 of them women, with a mean age of 62.3 years (Table 3.3). The cases were allotted to groups according to a predetermined statistically evaluated plan – twelve patients, six men and six women of comparable ages, were allotted to each of three groups and then given either 0.5 mg glucagon (Novo), 0.5 mg atropine, or a physiological saline solution as a placebo. The premedication was administered intravenously 5 minutes before endoscopy in the morning. The endoscopists did not know which premedication each patient had received, and the code was not broken before the study was finished. The patients' subjective complaints and the endoscopists' observations were immediately recorded on a scale line measuring 20 cm; the zero point indicated no complaints, and the 20 cm point the maximally pronounced complaints.

The results showed that there were no differences between glucagon and atropine concerning vomiting, opening of the pylorus, feeling of discomfort, or the estimated success of the examination (Table 3.4). Similarly, in these respects there were no differences between glucagon and atropine and the placebo. There was a significant difference, however, between glucagon and atropine concerning the estimates for peristalsis ($p = 0.002$) and reflux ($p = 0.006$) (Table 3.4). There were no differences between the two drugs where estimates of secretion of fluid and mucus were concerned, but both drugs showed effects which

TABLE 3.4 Comparison of the effect of glucagon with that of atropine. Significances indicated by p values

Findings	Glucagon	Atropine
Decrease in		
vomiting		0.36
secretion		0.37
salivation		0.29
inhibition of motility	0.002	
pyloric reflux	0.006	
pyloric opening		0.43
discomfort		0.46
Success of examination		0.49

were different from those of the placebo in this respect ($p = 0.02-0.03$).

In accordance with these results, a highly significant correlation was observed between the estimates for secretion and mucus production, and between reflux and peristalsis in all three groups (Tables 3.5 and 3.6). A partial correlation study showed that there were negative correlations between the size of the pylorus opening, and the vomiting and peristalsis in the three groups. (Tables 3.7–3.9.)

Conclusions from the above two studies

The conclusions from the above two studies are that glucagon is a valuable premedication for upper gastrointestinal endoscopy, and that it is superior to pethidine + atropine, and to atropine alone, when inhibition of peristalsis and pyloric reflux is desired. Such relaxation is needed for examination of the cause of

TABLE 3.5 Comparison of the effect of glucagon with that of a placebo. Significances indicated by p values

Findings	Glucagon	Placebo
Decrease in		
vomiting		0.21
secretion	0.02	
salivation	0.05	
inhibition of motility	0.0001	
pyloric reflux	0.002	
pyloric opening		0.30
discomfort		0.39
Success of examination		0.19

TABLE 3.6 Comparison of the effect of atropine with that of a placebo. Significances indicated by p values

Findings	Atropine	Placebo
Decrease in		
vomiting		0.36
secretion	0.03	
salivation		0.19
inhibition of motility		0.06
pyloric reflux		0.29
pyloric opening		0.48
discomfort		0.49
Success of examination		0.17

TABLE 3.7 Partial correlations (p values of r) in the placebo group

Observations	Vomit	Secretion	Salivation	Peristalsis	Pyl. reflux	Pyl. opening	Success	Discomfort
Vomiting	1	0.001	0.001	0.001		−0.001	−0.05	
Secretion		1	0.01	0.001		0.02	−0.001	
Salivation			1	0.005			−0.001	
Peristalsis, inhib.				1		−0.001		
Pyloric reflux					1	−0.05	−0.05	
Pyloric opening						1		0.05
Success of examination							1	
Discomfort								1

TABLE 3.8 Partial correlations (p values of r) in the glucagon group

Observations	Vomiting	Secretion	Salivation	Peristalsis	Pyl. reflux	Pyl. opening	Success	Discomfort
Vomiting	1			0.01	0.05	−0.001	−0.001	0.05
Secretion		1	0.001	0.001	0.001			
Salivation			1	0.05	0.01		−0.05	−0.05
Peristalsis, inhib.				1		−0.001	−0.001	0.001
Pyloric reflux					1	−0.05	−0.01	0.001
Pyloric opening						1	0.001	0.001
Success of examination							1	−0.001
Discomfort								1

TABLE 3.9 Partial correlations (p values of r) in the atropine group

Observations	Vomiting	Secretion	Salivation	Peristalsis	Pyl. reflux	Pyl. opening	Success	Discomfort
Vomiting	1	0.05	0.001			-0.05		0.01-
Secretion		1	0.001					-0.05
Salivation			1					0.05
Peristalsis, inhib.				1	0.01	-0.001		
Pyloric reflux					1	-0.001		
Pyloric opening						1		-0.05
Success of examination							1	
Discomfort								1

bleedings, small ulcers, and neoplasms, and when cannulation of the papilla of Vater with retrograde cholangio-pancreaticography is performed.

The role of glucagon in ERCP

The role of glucagon in ERCP has been compared to that of a glucose solution in a blind study involving 55 patients.[4] This study, in which other premedications were given along with the glucagon and the glucose solution, showed that a better relaxation of motility and an improved rate of success with less elevation of the urinary amylase values occurred when glucagon, rather than the glucose solution, was among the premedications given. Further studies, however, with more clearly defined groups, are needed before a firm conclusion can be drawn in this connection.

GLUCAGON AS PREMEDICATION FOR THERAPEUTIC PURPOSES

A beneficial effect of glucagon in patients subjected to gastric polypectomy has been reported by Hradsky and Furugaard,[14] but studies with control groups are needed before firm conclusions can be made. There is good reason to believe that glucagon would also be of benefit for papillotomy and in the treatment of biliary calculi, but, here again, controlled studies are needed in order that these suppositions can be confirmed.

CONCLUSIONS

The conclusion of this report, therefore, is that glucagon (Novo) serves as a good premedication in patients being subjected to endoscopic procedures of the upper gastrointestinal tract, particularly in cases involving bleedings or suspected small lesions. It is also reasonable to believe that glucagon is a suitable premedication for ERCP and papillotomy, as well as for polypectomy, but further research is needed before the final conclusion can be made on this point.

References

1 Bertrand, G., Woods, R. E., Raheja, K. L. and Linscheer, W. G. (1975). Double blind evaluation of two hypotonic drugs for duodenoscopy and duodenography. (Abstract) *Gastroenterology*, **68,** 1069.

2 Carsen, G. M. and Finby, N. (1976). Hypotonic duodenography with glucagon. *Radiology*, **118,** 529.

3 Chernish, S. M., Miller, R. E., Rosenak, B. D. and Scholz, N. E. (1972). Hypotonic duodenography with the use of glucagon. *Gastroenterology*, **63,** 392.

4 Silvis, S. E. and Vennes, J. A. (1975). The role of glucagon in endoscopic cholangiopancreatography. *Gastrointest. Endosc.*, **21,** 162.

5 Chernish, S. M., Miller, R. E., Rosenak, B. D. and Scholz, N. E. (1972). Effect of glucagon on size of visualized human gallbladder before and after a fat meal. *Gastroenterology*, **62,** 1218.

6 Paul, F. (1976). Intravenöse Langzeitinfusion von Glukagon zur Abtreibung von Gallenwegskonkrementen. *Fortschr. Endoskopie*, pp. 161–163. (Erlanger: Perimed).

7 Rey, J. F. and Harvey, R. F. (1977). Hormonal control of the sphincter of Oddi. In: *The Sphincter of Oddi* (J. Delmont, ed.). Proceedings, 3rd Gastroenterology Symp., Nice, 1976. pp. 66–71. (Basel: Karger).

8 Bernoulli, R., Faust, H., Gyr, K., Thurnherr, N., Aenishänslin, W. and Stalder, G. A. (1977). Prospektive studie der ersten 197 endoskopisch-retrograden Cholangiopankreatikographien (ERCP) Basel (1973–1975). *Schweiz. Med. Wochenschr.*, **107,** 1287.

9 Brandstätter, G. and Kratochvil, P. (1977). Anwendungmöglichkeiten von Glukagon im Bereich der gastrointestinalen Endoskopie. *Arch. Arzneitner.*, **1,** 172.

10 Hradsky, M., Stockbrügger, R. and Ostberg, H. (1973). The effect of glucagon on gastric motility, the pylorus and reflux of bile into the stomach during gastroscopic examination. (Abstract) *Scand. J. Gastroent.*, **8,** (suppl. 20), 26.

11 Hradsky, M., Stockbrügger, R., Dotevall, G. and Ostberg, H. (1973). The use of glucagon during upper gastrointestinal endoscopy. *Gastrointest. Endosc.*, **20,** 162.

12 Melsom, M., Myren, J., Larsen, S. and Moe, A. (1977). Comparison of glucagon and pethidine plus atropine as premedication for peroral endoscopy. *Endoscopy*, **9,** 79.

13 Qvigstad, T., Myren, J. and Larsen, S. (1978). Comparison of the effect of glucagon and atropine as premedication for endoscopy of the upper gastrointestinal tract. *Scand. J. Gastroenterol.* (In press).

14 Hradsky, M. and Furugaard, K. (1976). Electrosurgical gastric polypectomy and duodenoscopy with the use of glucagon Novo. *Scand. J. Gastroenterol.*, **11,** (Suppl. 38), 54.

DISCUSSION

McCarthy: We in Albuquerque have recently published on the control of upper gastrointestinal ulcer bleeding using endoscopic cauterization (Volpicelli, N.A. *et al.* (1978). *Arch. Surg.,* **113,** 483). It would seem, judging by what we have heard here, that glucagon tends to increase the splanchnic blood flow. That being true, would glucagon be inadvisable when one wishes to control gastrointestinal bleeding through cauterization, or when one is doing a papillotomy? Would the prospect of increased blood flow not lead to a greater likelihood of increased bleeding during such procedures?

Myren: I think you are probably right. It is true that glucagon increases blood flow in that area, and this would make it a little more dangerous for bleeders than for other patients. I think that a controlled study is needed of this aspect.

Wingate: The evidence from the literature is that glucagon increases splanchnic blood flow, but there is no evidence of what it does to mucosal blood flow. In other words, it might not be as dangerous as it sounds, certainly if one is not attempting anything too drastic.

Paul: Professor Myren, did you find that glucagon had an effect on the pyloric region? I have observed that the passage of endoscopic instruments through the pylorus is much easier after giving glucagon, and that in routine endoscopies of the upper gastrointestinal tract, including the oesophagus, the stomach, and the proximal duodenum, the procedure can be done much more quickly when this substance is given. It is the same with other spasmolytic agents. When you compared glucagon with placebo, did you record how quickly a routine procedure could be performed?

Myren: No, the time taken for endoscopy was not included in our parameters.

Volpicelli: One of the reasons for giving atropine, at least in my own practice, is to prevent vasovagal reactions. The second reason is to decrease salivary secretions. I did not understand exactly where you found a decrease in secretion.

Myren: We did not record the differing secretions in specific areas, but it is our impression that the secretions are decreased all over. As far as the effect on heart rhythm and vasovagal complications are concerned, we have done some 10 000 to 15 000 gastroscopies without encountering any serious problems.

Paul: I think you need not worry about vasovagal reactions. In about 10 000 endoscopies I have never observed a severe vasovagal reaction. To my mind, this potential problem is a bit over-estimated. I would like to make a comment on the action of glucagon on the pylorus, and to come back to species differences. In animal experiments Professor Halter from Berne, Switzerland, found that glucagon closes the pylorus. We, however, have never observed this effect in man.

Baker: I wonder, Professor Myren, if you would tell us about the diagnoses in these groups. I am surprised that with the better mucosal view you obtained in patients receiving glucagon, you were not able to establish a more precise diagnosis. I noticed, incidentally, that the patients were rather older than they would have been had the studies been done in our institution. Were the diagnoses similar in both groups?

Myren: There were no major differences in the diagnoses made in the two groups, but I think the groups were too small to answer this question about the ease of differentiating between various diseases.

Baker: The numbers were very small, I agree, but is it your impression that in a complicated patient, one for example with liver disease, oesophageal varices, gastritis, and a history of duodenal ulcer, glucagon would be of special help in establishing a firm diagnosis?

Myren: What I can say is that one certainly needs a quiet condition in order to be able to locate the lesions.

4 The Use of Glucagon in Colonoscopy

B. Ek

A study is currently being carried out in the Department of Medicine at the University of Umeå (Sweden) to test the value of glucagon as a premedication for colonoscopy.

The purpose of the present paper is to explain a little about the problems encountered during colonoscopy, and why it is expected that the Umeå study will show glucagon to be valuable as a premedication in this procedure.

FIBREOPTIC COLONOSCOPY

Fibreoptic techniques have been used in endoscopy for some 20 years.[1] The areas first studied by this means were the oesophagus, the stomach, and the upper part of the duodenum. In the Umeå clinic the first inspection of the colon with a fibreoptic endoscope, the fibrescope, was undertaken in 1971. The anatomy and the contents of the bowel caused many difficulties in the beginning, and even now anatomical variations and the physiological reactions of the bowel cause problems in individual cases.

The fibreoptic bundle consists of thousands of small glass fibres, each approximately 10-15 microns in diameter. The fibres, which are individually coated, are coherent, which means that they are similarly orientated at both ends and so permit the transmission of a visual image. Light is transmitted through the fibrescope to the tip from outside sources. Accessory channels are incorporated into the instrument to permit suction, insufflation, and the introduction of various instruments for the purpose of biopsy, etc. Wire equipment manipulated from the

53

ocular end of the fibrescope allows the tip to be deflected in any direction.

The colon is about 2 m long. Parts of it are attached to the highly mobile mesocolon; the result is a multitude of configurations in the colon, which is a cause of many difficulties during colonoscopy.

The main indications for colonoscopy are equivocal barium enema findings, unexplained bleedings and unexplained colonic symptoms, inflammatory bowel diseases, postoperative problems, and polypectomy.

Contraindications, provided that the patient is not critically ill, are few, but they include serious acute bouts of ulcerative colitis, Crohn's disease, ischaemic colitis, acute diverticulitis, infections, irradiation colitis, peritonitis, and pregnancy. Relative contraindications include frailty of the patient, previous pelvic operations or irradiation, and pendent sigma.

The preparation of the bowel is as follows:

1. A clear liquid diet for 2 days prior to the examination.
2. Laxatives (castor oil, magnesium sulphate) the evening before the colonoscopy.
3. Cleansing enemas (tap water, saline solution) early on the day of examination.

Premedication is often necessary, and, in order to make the colonoscopy more tolerable for the patient, analgesics are also often administered. It is, however, of immense importance that the patient remains able to register pain throughout the examination, and so aid the endoscopist. For this reason some authors recommend that premedication should not routinely be given.[2 3] In the Umeå clinic, where this examination is usually performed without the help of fluoroscopy, it has hitherto been usual to administer sedatives and analgesics. The medication normally given is 25–50 mg pethidine and 5–20 mg diazepam intravenously, the amounts depending on bodyweight. In spite of these drugs the patient has continued to be capable of recognizing undue pain and of informing the endoscopist. An anticholinergic, 0.5 mg atropine intramuscularly, is also usually given before the examination in order to abolish contractions and peristalsis, and, if necessary, this is given again during the examination.

The intubation of the instrument is performed with the patient in the left lateral position. The fibrescope is inserted into the colon and, with the help of tip deflection, the instrument bowing and torqueing, air insufflation, and water cleansing, and of such specialized techniques as the slide-by, the alfa manoeuvre, and hooking-lifting-telescoping, the splenic flexure can be reached in about 90% of cases[4] and the caecum in 75–83%.

The amount of time required to perform a colonoscopy varies from several minutes to some hours.

With the use of forceps, brushes, and flexible snares, it is possible to obtain samples for histopathological studies, and to perform therapeutic polypectomies.

Complications may occur, but these are few in experienced hands. The most serious risk is that of bowel perforation. In a survey of 1106 colonoscopy cases, a perforation incidence of 0.9% was observed.[5] Other complications reported include retroperitoneal emphysema,[6] the tearing of the mesosigmoid,[7] and the serosal tearing of the sigmoid.[4]

In the Umeå clinic upper gastrointestinal endoscopies have been performed since 1962 and colonoscopies since 1971. As in other hospitals,[8] each year since then there has been a great increase in the number of endoscopies performed. This trend will continue, and as it does, so the need for the examinations to be performed more efficiently and speedily, and so less expensively, will increase.

Hypermotility of the gastrointestinal tract is often a problem in endoscopic examinations. The administration of anticholinergic drugs to treat hypermotility, smooth muscle spasm and vasovagal reflexes has been recommended,[9 10] but the adverse effects of these drugs mean that their use cannot be recommended in all cases, certainly not in older patients nor in those who may be suffering from glaucoma, prostatism, tachyarrythmia, or cardioarteriosclerosis.

THE USE OF GLUCAGON

The use of glucagon to decrease the tone and contractions of the upper gastrointestinal tract during radiological[11-14] and endoscopic examinations[14-1] has been reported as valuable, though reports on controlled studies are few.[14 17]

Although the effect of glucagon on gastrointestinal motility was early recognized in the colon of the dog, interest in its use in colonic examinations in man has been small until recently.

Glucagon has, however, now been advocated as a safe hypomotility drug in barium enema studies of the colon.[13 18-20]

In controlled studies it has produced significantly less discomfort for the patient and better diagnostic films for the radiologist than placebo.[13 19-21] With glucagon the colon has been seen to be more relaxed, the intracolonic pressure less, and the intensity and number of side effects smaller than with atropine.[13] The reported side effects are nausea, profuse perspiration, vertigo, and headache,[12-14 18 22 23] but most authors describe the incidence of these complaints as being low, and not significantly higher than seen when a placebo is administered.[21] Some, however, have found the incidence of side effects to be higher with glucagon than with atropine.[23]

There are a few reports on the use of glucagon as a pharmacological adjunct to colonoscopy.[14 24] The dose of glucagon was 0.2–1 mg intravenously, the effect was nearly instantaneous and lasted for between 10 and 20 min.

Experience in the Umeå clinic has shown glucagon to be successful in connection with oesophago-gastroduodenoscopy, and it was partly this which led to the consideration of its use as a hypomotility drug in connection with colonoscopy.

For practical and economic reasons colonoscopy is performed without the help of fluoroscopy in the Umeå clinic, which means that some colonoscopies have to be repeated before the desired information is obtained. Functional disorders are very common in the colon. An irritable colon *per se*, or one complicating another organic disorder, often causes problems in colonoscopy, and the spasms occurring in such cases cannot always be successfully overcome with anticholinergics.

For the past year glucagon has also been used successfully

in the Umeå clinic as a hypotonic agent in lower gastro-intestinal endoscopies, and the results obtained here also in-dicated its likely usefulness in colonoscopy.

Before carrying out the present study a small pilot study was conducted. This involved 13 patients, and was a com-parative test between glucagon and placebo. In all instances, glucagon was found to permit total colonoscopy, i.e., an ex-amination of the entire colon, to be performed more speedily and with much less discomfort to the patient.

References

1 Hirschowitz, B. I., Curtiss, L. E., Peters, C. W. *et al.* (1958). Demonstration of a new gastroscope "Fiberscope". *Gastroenterology*, **30**, 50.
2 Deyhle, P. and Demling, L. (1971). Coloscopy – technique, results, in-dications. *Endoscopy*, **3**, 143.
3 Williams, C. B. and Muto, T. (1972). Examination of the whole colon with fibreoptic colonoscope. *Br. Med. J.*, **3**, 278.
4 Overholt, B. F. (1975). Colonoscopy – a review. *Gastroenterology*, **68**, 1308.
5 Geenen, J. E., Schmitt, W. G. Jr. and Hogan, W. J. (1974). Complications of
. colonoscopy. *Gastrointest. Endosc.*, **66**, 812.
6 Lezak, M. B. and Goldhamer, M. (1974). Retroperitoneal emphysema after colonoscopy. *Gastroenterology*, **66**, 118.
7 Fox, J. A. (1972). Fibreoptic colonoscopy. *Proc. Soc. Med.*, **65**, 38.
8 Schiller, K. F. R. (1973). The growth in gastrointestinal endoscopy. Memorandum on future national needs for fibre-optic endoscopy of the gastrointestinal tract. *Br. Soc. Digest. Endosc.* September.
9 Welin, S. (1958). Modern trends in diagnostic roentgenology of the colon. *Br. J. Radiol.*, **31**, 453.
10 Ferrucci, J. T. Jr. and Benedict, K. T. Jr. (1971). Anticholinergic-aided study of the gastrointestinal tract. *Radiol. Clin. North Am.*, **9**, 23.
11 Necheles, H., Sporn, J. and Walker, L. (1966). Effect of glucagon on gastro-intestinal motility. *Am. J. Gastroenterol.*, **45**, 34.
12 Chernish, S. M., Miller, R. E., Rosenak, B. D. and Scholz, N. E. (1972). Hypotonic duodenography with the use of glucagon. *Gastroenterology*, **63**, 392.
13 Miller, R. E., Chernish, S. M., Skucas, J., Rosenak, B. D. and Rodda, B. E. (1974). Hypotonic colon examination with glucagon. *Radiology*, **113**, 555.
14 Paul, F. and Freyschmidt, J. (1976). Anwendung von Glukagon bei en-doskopischen und röntgenologischen Untersuchungen des Gastro-intestinaltrackts. *Fortschr. Geb. Roentgenstr.*, **125**, 31.
15 Hradsky, M., Stockbrügger, R. and Ostberg, H. (1973). The effect of glucagon on gastric motility, the pylorus and reflux of bile into the stomach

during gastroscopic examination. (Abstract) *Scand. J. Gastroenterol.* **8** (suppl. 20), 26.

16 Paul, F., Misaki, F. and Seifert, E. (1973). Crystalline pancreatic glucagon – a new spasmolytic agent: results of comparative endoscopic and electromanometric investigations in the proximal gastrointestinal tract. *Endoscopy*, **5**, 199.

17 Melsom, M., Myren, J., Larsen, S. and Moe, A. (1977). Comparison of glucagon and pethidine plus atropine as premedication for peroral endoscopy. *Endoscopy*, **9**, 79.

18 Gohel, V. K., Dalinka, M. K. and Coren, G. S. (1975). Hypotonic examination of the colon with glucagon. *Radiology*, **115**, 1.

19 Meeroff, J. C., Jorgens, J. and Isenberg, J. I. (1975). The effect of glucagon on barium enema examination. *Radiology*, **115**, 5.

20 Taylor, I., Duthie, H. L., Cumberland, D. C. and Smallwood, R. (1975). Glucagon and the colon. *Gut*, **16**, 973.

21 Harned, R. K., Stelling, C. B., Williams, S. and Wolf, G. L. (1976). Glucagon and barium enema examinations – a controlled clinical trial. *Am. J. Roentgenol.*, **126**, 981.

22 Jerell, J. J. (1976). Use of glucagon as the hypotonic agent in barium enema examination. *J. Am. Osteopath. Assoc.*, **76**, 264.

23 Poser, H. and Baier, J. (1977). Vergleichende pharmako-dynamische Kolon-Doppelkontrastuntersuchung mit Glukagon und Atropin. *Radiol. Diagnost.*, **18**, 355.

24 Brandstätter, G. and Kratochvil, P. (1977). Anwendungsmöglichkeiten von Glukagon im Bereich der gastrointestinalen Endoskopie. *Arch. Arzneitner.*, **1**, 172.

DISCUSSION

Myren: Are you planning to give both diazepam and glucagon to the patients in your study? In my experience, though we rarely give premedication for colonoscopy, only when a patient is extremely nervous, the effects of these two substances are so similar that it would be difficult if you gave both to see which were the results of the diazepam and which were attributable to glucagon. Your study would probably be more useful if you could have three groups: one on glucagon, one on diazepam, and one on placebo.

Ek: All the colonoscopies I have done have been in patients premedicated with low doses of diazepam, and it seemed reasonable not to change the routine when doing this study. Each of the patients in the study is his own control, and one is able to compare the effect of glucagon with that of placebo as diazepam is given with both.

Volpicelli: A negative report on a study rather similar to the one you are planning has recently been published (Norfleet, R.G. (1978). *Gastrointestinal Endoscopy,* **24,** 164). In this study there was no benefit for either the performance of colonoscopy or the comfort of the patient. My own experience is that the actual insertion of the scope is more difficult once stasis is produced, since, once the colon is paralyzed, one cannot make use of the intrinsic motor activity in order to 'shorten the colon'. There are, however, a number of patients, those with spastic colons for example, in whom the induction of stasis permits a more complete examination of the colon. For this purpose glucagon is certainly the best substance I have found.

Paul: You mentioned, Professor Ek, that you usually perform colonoscopy without using fluoroscopy. Personally, I would have thought this rather unwise, as, without some sort of X-ray control, one can never be certain of where one is. After inserting the endoscope $1\frac{1}{2}$ metres one may indeed have reached the caecum, but one may also still be in the sigmoid colon. The sigmoid is sometimes very mobile, and in these cases it can easily be pushed up to the splenic flexure or even to the transverse colon.

Myren: Yes, I agree with that.

Wingate: The value of glucagon in these situations seems to me to be that if injected intravenously it has a very reliable relaxant effect on the gut. My feeling is that it is invaluable when one wants just a brief period of relaxation, but a fully conscious patient. Once one starts using sedation or anaesthesia the situation becomes very much more complicated. Glucagon makes the examination easier, safer for the patient, and probably quicker too.

I am a little concerned, Professor Ek, that you include 'unexplained colonic symptoms' as an indication for colonoscopy, a procedure which you say has a 1% serious complications rate. How does one know when a problem comes from the colon?

Ek: At my hospital we have to deal with problem cases sent from other hospitals in northern Sweden. In these cases there is often concern about the state of the colon. Before one can diagnose irritable colon in these cases, one has to rule out organic lesions, and this is done with colonoscopy.

5 Glucagon in Radiology

L. Kreel

Pharmacoradiology is now widely accepted. There was, quite rightly, an initial resistance due to unpredictable results and the unacceptable incidence of side effects. Morphine, insulin and prostigmine were rapidly discarded and replaced by metoclopramide, propantheline and hyoscine butyl bromide. These substances are highly effective and, while the side effects are predictable and acceptable, the incidence of side effects of propantheline is nevertheless quite high.

In the last decade quality control in radiology has been emphasized particularly to show greater detail. In gastrointestinal radiology this has led to the use of double contrast techniques, where drugs are absolutely essential for the quality of the examination and in the barium enema also for the comfort of the patient. The safety of glucagon, its freedom from side effects, rapidity of action and reliability have resulted in its widespread acceptance. The mitigating factors are cost and availability. There has, however, been no determined campaign to reduce the cost and conserve world supplies by the use of minimal effective doses. Radiologists are now among the major users of this drug and should be fully aware of its indications, limitations, length of action, route of administration, possible side effects and contra-indications.

ACTION OF GLUCAGON RELEVANT TO RADIOLOGY[1] (Table 5.1)

Glucagon appears to act directly on smooth muscle rather than by neuromuscular transmission and probably produces its effect by enhancing adenyl cyclase activity.[2] Late effects may occur

TABLE 5.1 Pharmacological effects of glucagon

Stimulation

1. Renal excretion of electrolytes
2. Increase in cardiac output
3. Release of growth hormone
4. Bronchodilation
5. Release of insulin
6. Increase in serum lipids
7. Increase in biliary flow

Inhibition

1. Reduction of pancreatic secretion
2. Reduction of HCl and peptic gastric secretion
3. Reduction of basal and gastrin-induced mucosal blood flow
4. Reduction of gastric motility
5. Reduction of intestinal motility
6. Relaxation of the gallbladder

From Meeroff *et al.* (1975)[1]

due to stimulation of insulin production. Glucagon also produces renal excretion of electrolytes and increased bile flow.

However, from the radiological viewpoint its main action is in diminishing the tone and motility of stomach, duodenum, small bowel and colon, thus abolishing peristalsis and allowing full distension. It has no effect on oesophageal peristalsis but does relax the cardiac sphincter or oesophago-gastric junction. Glucagon probably also relaxes the ureteric and bladder smooth muscle as well as arterioles, and has a similar action on the gall bladder as well as the sphincter of Oddi but in doses much smaller than cholecystokinin.[3 4] Further effects which may be relevant to gastrointestinal radiology are the reduction in hydrochloric acid and peptic gastric secretion associated with both basal and gastrin-induced gastric mucosal blood flow. There is also a reduction of exocrine pancreatic secretion.

DOSAGE AND ROUTE OF ADMINISTRATION
Glucagon is unfortunately inactivated when given orally but is

effective both intravenously and intramuscularly. By intravenous injection its effects are virtually instantaneous coming on in 15–30 seconds. 0.1 mg is an effective dose for barium meal, duodenal and colonic studies, but most workers use 0.2–0.25 mg. The usual intramuscular dose, 0.75–1.5 mg. starts acting in 5–15 minutes and its action persists for 30–60 minutes. The intravenous route is thus ideal for gastrointestinal barium examinations particularly as it does not interfere with gastric emptying because its action wears off so rapidly. There is also a suggestion that the 'insulin rebound' activity aids in the demonstration of the small bowel by causing intestinal hurry. The terminal ileum can subsequently be shown in the vast majority of cases in 30–60 minutes.[5] The more prolonged action of intramuscular glucagon is an advantage in computed tomography where aperistalsis is required for examinations of the abdomen and examinations last $\frac{1}{2}$–1 hour.[6]

SIDE EFFECTS[5 7-10]

With small intravenous doses of 0.1–0.25 mg side effects are virtually unknown,[5 11] apart from those associated with the injection itself or the ingestion of barium. Thus occasional patients may have a vaso-vagal attack or vomiting. With doses of 1–2 mg, vomiting, nausea, dizziness, flushing, dry mouth and diarrhoea have been reported but considerably less than with propantheline. Nausea and vomiting often come on 1–2 hours after the injection and last 5–10 minutes. However, no serious complications such as gastric dilatation or inconvenient complications such as urinary retention have been reported.[7-9]

CONTRA-INDICATIONS

There are virtually no contra-indications to glucagon when given in diagnostic radiology in minimum doses of 0.1–0.2 mg intravenously. For larger doses the possibility of provoking reactive hypoglycaemia in patients with insulinoma and hypertension in phaeochromocytoma patients must be considered and is particularly relevant to computed tomography examinations of the suprarenal. The possibility of hypersensitivity exists but no valid report associated with diagnostic radiology is available in the literature although insulin as a contaminant has been implicated.[12-13] When the suprarenals are being investigated with computed tomography to exclude a phaeochromocytoma, it is advisable to use propantheline or hyoscine butyl bromide rather than glucagon.

INDICATIONS IN RADIODIAGNOSIS (Table 5.2)

Glucagon is mainly used in gastrointestinal radiology and

TABLE 5.2 Indications for glucagon in radiodiagnosis

1. Barium swallow
2. Barium meal
3. Duodenography
4. Small bowel
5. Bile ducts and gallbladder
6. Barium enema
7. Endoscopy
8. Arteriography
9. Hysterosalpingography
10. Urography
11. Computed tomography

endoscopy for examination of the stomach, duodenum and colon. In diagnostic radiology the rationale depends on overwhelming evidence of the greater reliability and accuracy of double contrast barium examinations. Endoscopy is also largely concerned with the stomach, duodenum and colon. With the advent of computed tomography, glucagon has found another indispensable role in diagnostic radiology. In the oesophagus and biliary system, in arteriography, urography and hysterosalpingography its indications are considerably less, but for the sake of completeness will be included.

GASTROINTESTINAL RADIOLOGY

Barium swallow (Figure 5.1)

No absolute indications are available for the use of glucagon in

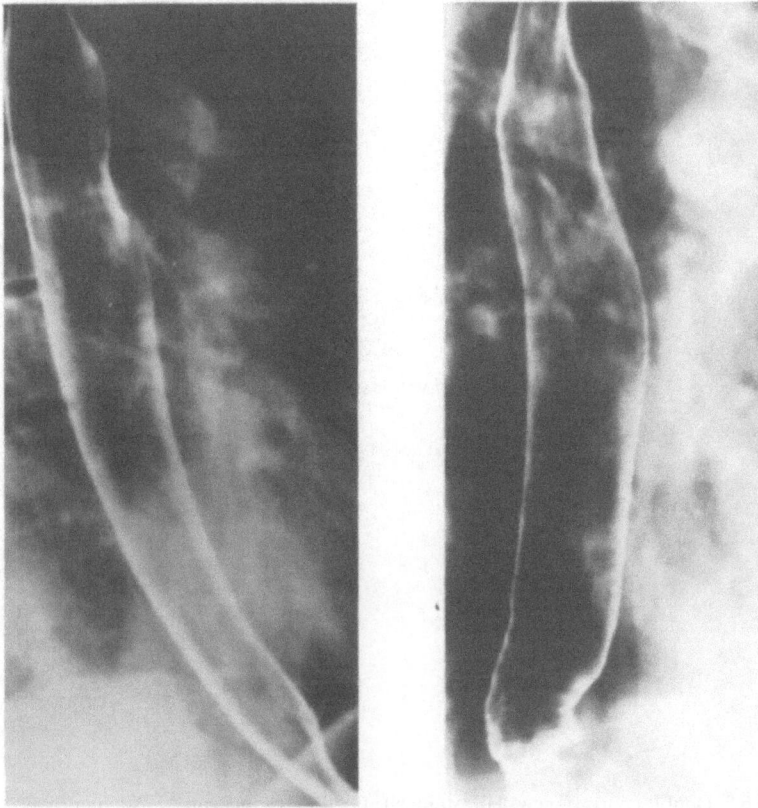

Figure 5.1 Normal double contrast barium swallows. 0.1 mg of glucagon i.v. was given for the barium meal examination. Glucagon has no effect on oesophageal peristalsis but does not interfere with the visualization

the oesophagus but equally there are no contra-indications. The absence of contra-indications is particularly relevant because the oesophagus is routinely examined in barium meal examinations. If reflux or hiatus hernia were hidden or provoked then the use of glucagon would clearly need to be questioned.

For the demonstration of varices, hyoscine butyl bromide and propantheline[14-17] have been shown to be valuable, but not glucagon; probably because glucagon does not inhibit oesophageal peristalsis. However, glucagon does relax the oesophageal sphincter.[10 18] Thus in cases of achalasia[19] it produces lowering of sphincteric pressure, and may be used to

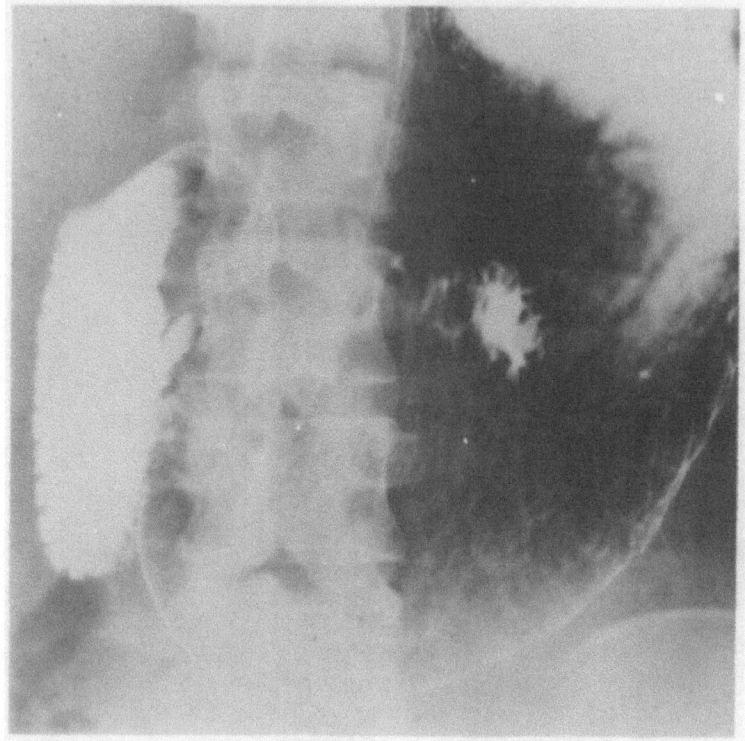

Figure 5.2 Double contrast view of the stomach after 0.1 mg glucagon i.v. Adequate gas distension following myorelaxant effect

disimpact a food bolus[20] or relieve spasm of the cardia associated with reflux, especially in the post-operative period.

The barium meal (Figure 5.2, 5.3)

Gastric atony is an essential part of the modern technique of double contrast barium meal examination[21 22] and glucagon has been used in small doses by intravenous injection since 1974. It is possible that glucagon is such an effective agent in the double contrast barium meal not only because of its action in relaxing the smooth muscle but also because it diminishes hydrochloric acid and peptic gastric secretions[23] allowing better visualization of areae gastricae and small surface lesions such as gastric erosions, polyps, ulcer scars and early gastric cancer.

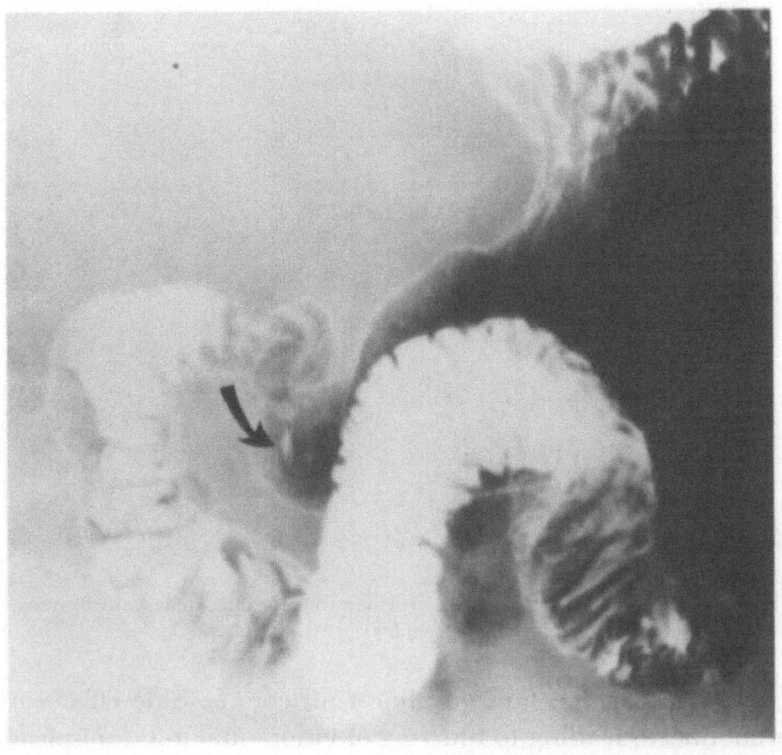

Figure 5.3 Small slit ulcer in gastric antrum (0.1 mg glucagon i.v.)

The use of any agent in radiology will stand or fall by its efficacy in the most common examinations. It is therefore important to assess its place in barium meals and to compare it with other agents. In double contrast barium meals the stomach must be atonic long enough to show all its parts. Initially, the barium must remain in the stomach so that the third part of the duodenum does not superimpose on the stomach.[24] Thereafter, the pylorus must be sufficiently open for barium and air to pass into the duodenum (Figures 5.4, 5.5), which must still be relaxed for a 'tubeless' duodenogram to be done. Should a follow-through examination be required the drug used must not prolong the transit through the small bowel, and finally the side effects must be minimal and inconsequential.

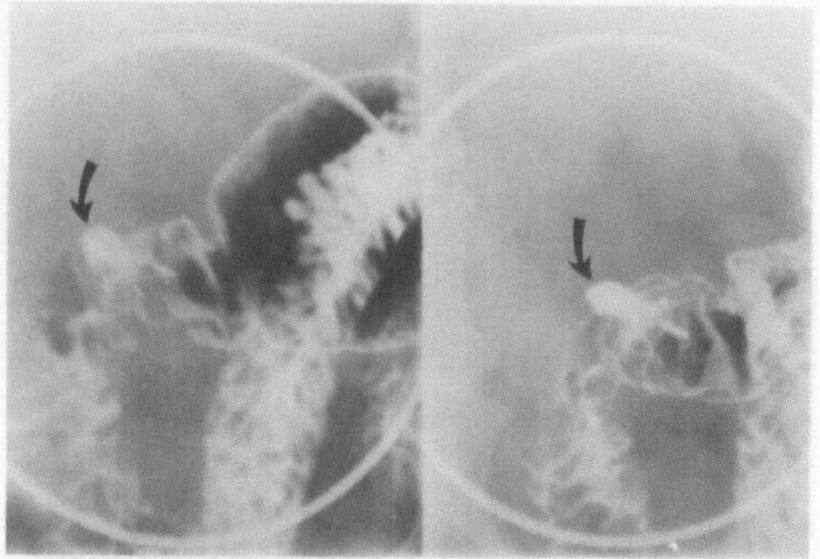

Figure 5.4 Duodenal relaxation helps to demonstrate the duodenal ulcer which shows barium retention (arrow) (0.1 mg glucagon i.v.)

Propantheline fails on almost all counts. Side effects are pronounced, leading to blurring of vision, making it unsafe for many patients to drive themselves. Urinary retention often occurs and gastric dilatation has been reported. Should a follow-through be required the barium transit through the small bowel is markedly prolonged which usually means that this part of the examination must be done separately.

The short-acting anticholinergics such as oxyphenonium bromide and hyoscine butyl bromide were thus a great advance. The side effects are less pronounced but blurred vision lasting 2–6 hours is not uncommon and urinary retention occasional. There is also some prolongation of barium transit through the intestine. The advantage of glucagon is that it is virtually free of side effects and, as an intravenous injection of 0.1–0.25 mg, does not interfere with transit through the small bowel. Hyoscine butyl bromide and glucagon would otherwise appear to be of equal value in the double contrast examination of the stomach, the former being somewhat cheaper compared with 0.1–0.2 mg glucagon.

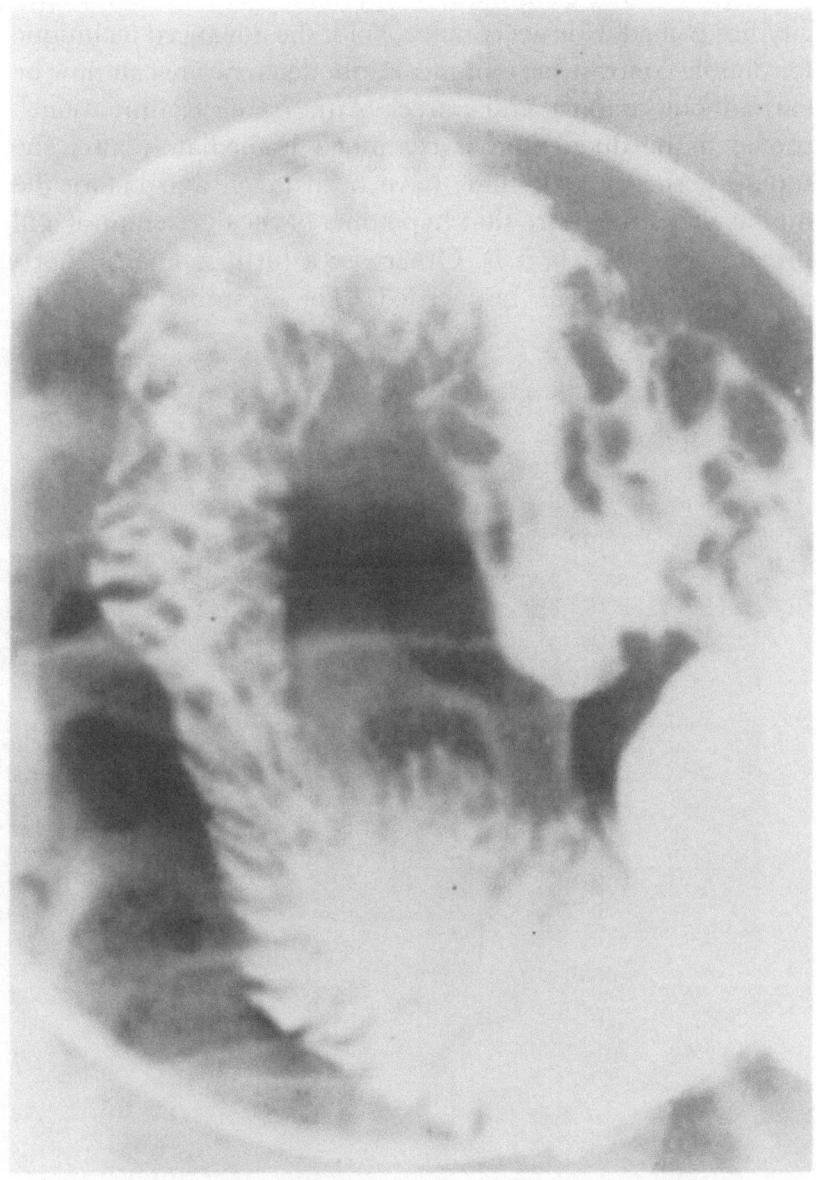

Figure 5.5 Hypertrophied Brunner's glands. Moderate duodenal relaxation about 10 minutes after 0.1 mg glucagon i.v.

The duodenogram

Initially, detailed examinations of the duodenum were performed using a tube[25][26] and a double contrast technique,[27] but later as a tubeless examination[28][29] which because of its simplicity has gained wide acceptance. With the advanced technique for double contrast barium meals, duodenography can now be carried out as part and parcel of the same examination,[30] provided the duodenum is examined immediately after the supine posterior wall films have been taken and before the fundus views to ensure that hypotonia of the duodenum is still present (Figures 5.6, 5.7). Otherwise a further dose of short-acting relaxant will be needed. The examination of the

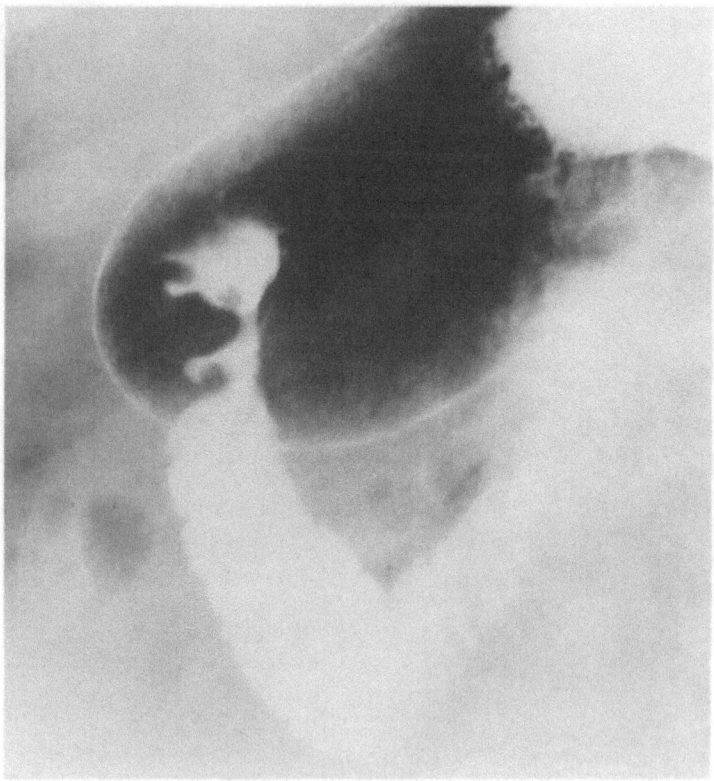

Figure 5.6 Post-bulbar duodenal ulceration. Relaxed duodenum with 0.1 mg glucagon i.v.

duodenum must not be delayed for another reason as well: returning barium-filled loops of jejunum will obscure the lower part of the duodenal sweep. Neither hyoscine butyl bromide nor glucagon has been shown to interfere in any way with barium coating of the duodenum[31] although there are reports that glucagon stimulates secretion from Brunner's glands in duodenal pouches of dogs.[32]

The 'post-operative stomach' (excluding immediate post-operative period)

The radiological examination of the post-operative stomach presents a real challenge. The small capacity of the gastric

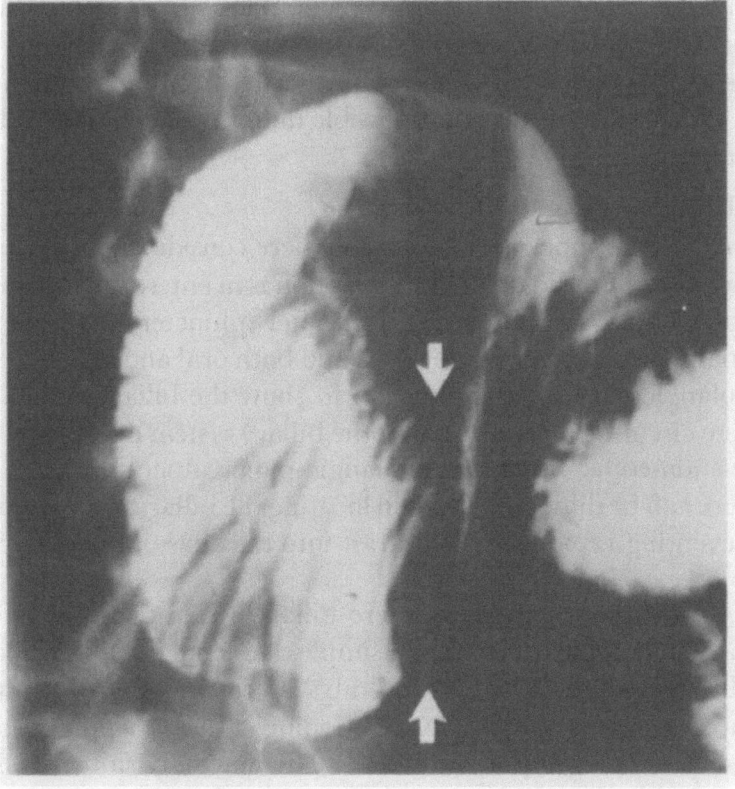

Figure 5.7 Marked duodenal relaxation associated with superior mesenteric artery 'compression' of third part of duodenum (arrows)

remnant after polya-type gastrectomies and the rapid exodus of barium and gas from the stomach make it difficult to obtain adequate distention and 'coating'. Furthermore, it is imperative to examine adequately both the afferent and efferent loops as well as the stoma after any form of gastroenterostomy, and for these reasons spasmolytic drugs are essential in barium examinations, especially to fill the afferent loop.[33] Somewhat more prolonged atony is required and therefore 0.25–0.5 mg of glucagon is recommended for late post-gastrectomy barium meal examinations, particularly if there is any question of excluding functional 'obstruction'.

With the use of gastric atony the afferent loop can almost invariably be filled with barium in the prone oblique position. Then, by turning the patient into the supine position, gas will enter the afferent loop to produce a double contrast view. In any case being investigated for malabsorption after gastrectomy or gastroenterostomy a 'blind loop' causing intestinal stasis must be excluded, and this is not possible unless the afferent loop has been shown.

Bile ducts and gall bladder

Another post-operative situation where considerable difficulty may arise in radiological investigation is in entero-biliary communications, or to a lesser extent after sphincterotomy. Gas is usually present in the bile ducts and both oral and intravenous cholangiography invariably fail to show the biliary system in these circumstances. Although the biliary system may be shown by endoscopic retrograde cholangio-pancreatography (ERCP) there can be difficulties both in locating the biliary orifice and in preventing rapid spill of contrast into the anastomosed loop of bowel.

The 'post-operative' entero-biliary system can be shown using spasmolytics by either a simple duodenal tube, a balloon-tube technique,[34] or by a 'tubeless' technique. With the 'tubeless' technique gravity-positioning of the patient is needed after producing hypotonia of the duodenum for barium to reflux into the bile duct. Subsequently, gas distension of the duodenum allows gas to enter the bile duct and produces a double contrast examination of the entero-biliary region to show the relevant anatomy. Both hyoscine butyl bromide and glucagon are effective in this examination.

In T-tube and intra-operative cholangiography, glucagon can be used to overcome any delay in passage of contrast into the duodenum due to muscle contraction[35] (Figure 5.8), and is particularly valuable in distinguishing organic fibrotic stenosis from 'spasm', bearing in mind the choloretic effect of glucagon.[36] Thus glucagon has been found effective in treatment of biliary colic and in facilitating spontaneous passage of common bile duct stones.[63]

Another important use of glucagon is in the non-operative extraction of biliary calculi both by the percutaneous route[35] and during endoscopic sphincterotomy. However the action on the sphincter of Oddi appears to be biphasic with initial contraction lasting 1–2 minutes before the myorelaxant action supervenes.

Glucagon relaxes the gall bladder making the gall bladder shadow larger if given both before and after a fatty meal,[37] but with a fatty meal given after glucagon the gall bladder is larger than if glucagon is given before the fatty meal.

The small bowel

For the small bowel enema, which is the recommended method of examination, spasmolytic drugs are not required. For routine follow-through examinations after a barium meal/duodeno-gram, the important feature is to see that transit through the small bowel is reasonably rapid, that the barium does not flocculate or segment, and that a small number of films can be taken to show the whole of the small bowel. Most spasmolytic drugs including 1–2 mg intramuscular glucagon thus interfere with the follow-through examination, but not 0.1–0.2 mg intravenous glucagon, and if anything the rebound 'insulin' effect increases barium transit through the small bowel.[38]

The barium enema

The barium enema is for the patient one of the more uncomfortable examinations and for the radiologist one of the most difficult to perform adequately. Spasmolytic drugs are used

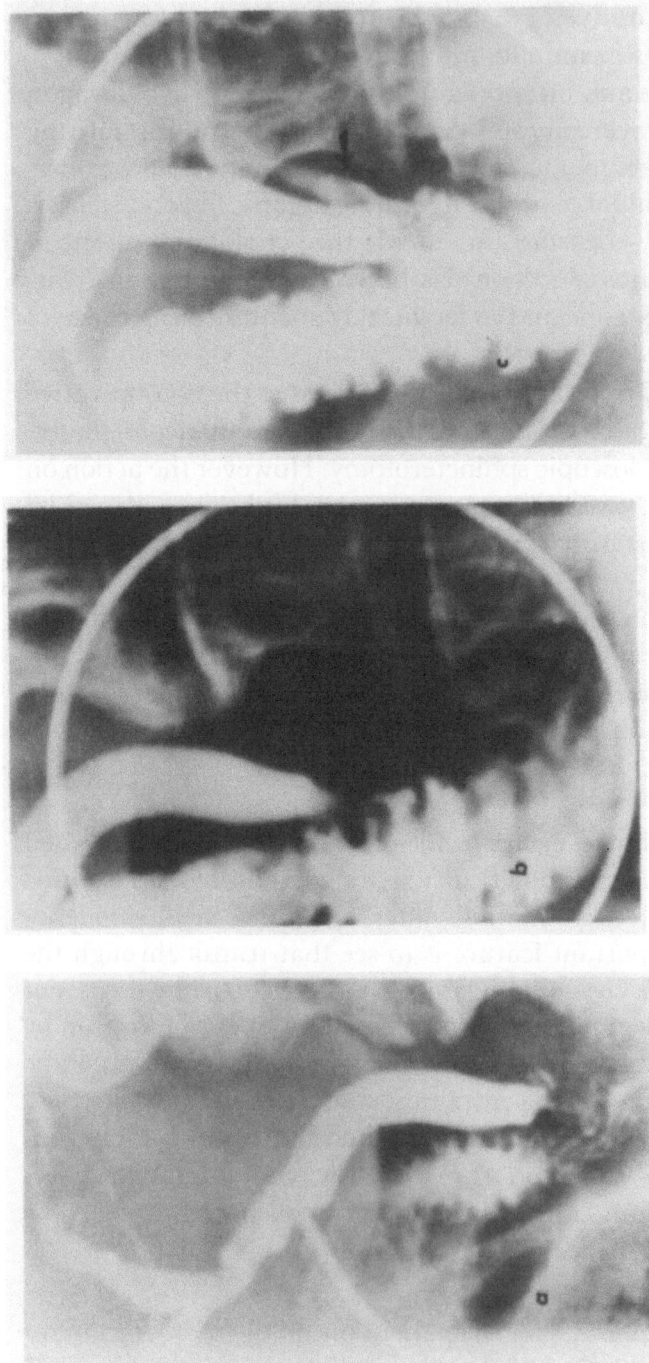

Figure 5.8 T-tube cholangiogram. (a) 'Shouldering' effect at distal end of common bile duct. (b) Two minutes after 0.25 mg glucagon i.v. showing relaxed distal end of common bile duct and duodenum. (c) After five minutes reflux into Wirsung's duct with small 'filling defect' in it (arrow)

routinely in the double contrast technique,[39][40] usually as oral medication some 30–60 minutes prior to the examination. If during the procedure an area of narrowing is detected or there is hold up of barium, intravenous hyoscine butyl bromide is usually given and subsequently glucagon has been recommended.[9-41] It has also been suggested as routine in barium enemas to make the examination more comfortable and decrease filling time to the caecum.[42]

Glucagon should particularly be used when there is diffuse painful spasm as in ulcerative or granulomatous colitis and in functional disorders, to evaluate areas of localized narrowing. in diverticular disease, and in the elderly when there is difficulty in retaining the barium,[9][43] but there is a good case for its routine use in a dose of 0.1–0.2 mg for the double contrast barium enema. Glucagon has also been recommended as an aid in barium enema reduction of intussusception.[44] The usual precautions must, of course, be taken, especially not using a hydrostatic pressure of more than 76 cm (30 in). There may be an increased incidence of ileal reflux of barium which has been claimed as interfering with colonic visualization,[45] but even if it was shown that ileal reflux occurs more frequently this could be an advantage in demonstrating the terminal ileum.

ENDOSCOPY

The reasons for the use of spasmolytics in endoscopy, whether for the stomach, duodenum or colon, are essentially similar to those in barium examinations. Unlike barium examinations most patients for endoscopy already get atropine 0.5 mg subcutaneously and 5–10 mg diazepam (Valium) intravenously.[49] With the stomach fully relaxed the mucosal folds become flattened allowing a better view of the gastric surface. This is important not only for diagnosis and gastrocamera filming but also for taking biopsies,[47] polypectomy[46] and even the removal of foreign bodies.[48]

It has been recommended that if glucagon·is used for ERCP it should be given only after the pylorus is negotiated,[50] but other workers suggest that it is easier to negotiate the pylorus after glucagon.[63] The advantage of glucagon over other spasmolytics is similar to that for its use in radiology. There are virtually no side effects, but when these are present they are less severe, less common, and last only for a short while.[51] Complications associated with ERCP are largely due to over-injection producing parenchymal filling, and when obviated the complication rate drops markedly,[52] although there has been a report of a significant reduction in the frequency and magnitude of urinary amylase after the use of glucagon.[53]

In endoscopy of the colon, relaxation is as important if not more so than in examinations of the stomach and duodenum and there is also no objection to repeated doses of 0.1–0.2 mg intravenously should movements return.

HYSTEROSALPINGOGRAPHY

It is not uncommon during hysterosalpingography for apparent obstruction to the flow of contrast to occur which can be relieved by a spasmolytic to produce free contrast spill onto the peritoneum showing duct patency.[54] Intravenous hyoscine butyl bromide has been used for this purpose but recently glucagon has also been shown to be effective.[55]

ARTERIOGRAPHY

Injected glucagon can produce a 50% increase in hepatic blood flow[56], and also causes increased blood flow when given directly into the superior mesenteric artery.[57] When used in arteriography it produces better opacification of the terminal branches with a more intense blush in both coeliac and mesenteric artery injections.[58]

UROLOGY

In the kidney glucagon causes a definite increase in renal blood flow and has a prolonged effect with an increase in the measured diameter of arteries, but without a change in the nephrographic effect or venous phase,[59] indicating that it does not cause pre-glomerular shunting. There is also a suggestion that glucagon causes relaxation of the ureter with easier passage of calculi,[60] and it is certainly known that glucagon causes renal excretion of electrolytes.[61] There is also a suggestion that it causes some relaxation of the bladder.

COMPUTED TOMOGRAPHY (Figure 5.9)

From the outset it was clear that the best results in body CT would only be produced if there was attention to detail and careful patient preparation and management.[62] Computed tomography is by no means an automated process and one of the major concerns is the control of bowel movements to minimize streak artefacts. Initially, intramuscular propantheline was used because of its prolonged action but due to the common occurrence of side effects, particularly in the elderly, every effort is being made to use other substances. At present intravenous glucagon is extensively used, given in doses of 0.25-0.5 mg intravenously, but recently the regime has been changed to 1 mg intramuscularly and 0.25 mg intravenously. The major side effect with this dose in the occasional patient is a single loose

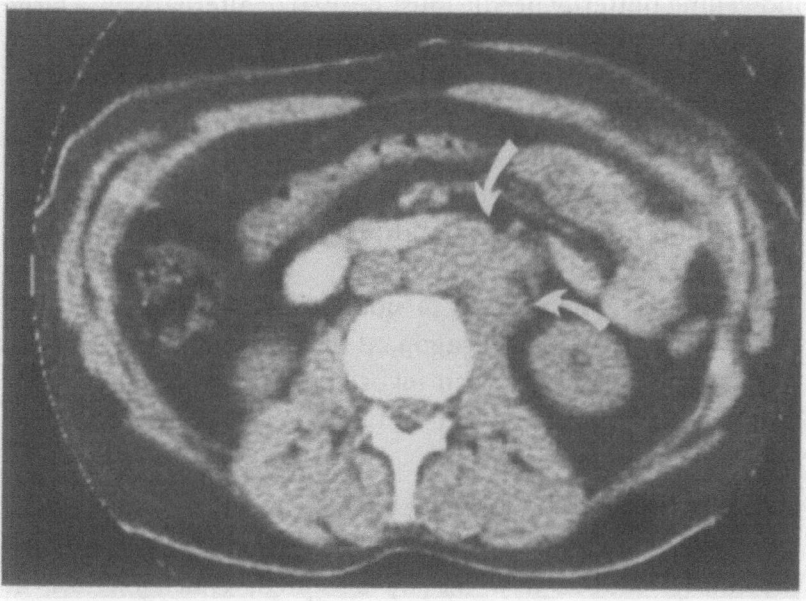

Figure 5.9 Computed tomography with scan time of 20 seconds. Movement free with no artefacts from colon or small bowel in spite of gas and contrast. Lymphadenopathy in the left para-aortic region (arrow)

bowel action, and transient nausea may also occur. It is in CT, because of its ability to demonstrate the suprarenals clearly, that one must be particularly aware of phaeochromocytomas as being a contra-indication to the use of glucagon.

Glucagon undoubtedly diminishes bowel movements and streak artefacts in scanners having an 18-20 second scan time but its exact role in devices with short scanning times of 3-6 seconds remains to be seen.

DISADVANTAGES OF GLUCAGON

The two major disadvantages of glucagon have now largely been overcome. There is no longer a shortage of world supply and when used in its minimum effective dose it is comparable in price to anticholinergic drugs such as hyoscine butyl bromide. In the double contrast barium meal as little as 0.1-0.2 mg, given intravenously, is effective. However repeated injections are unacceptable to both patients and radiologists. Where a prolonged effect is required, as with computed tomography, an indwelling butterfly needle must be used or alternatively a large dose given intramuscularly, such as 1 mg with a loading dose of 0.25 mg intravenously. The minor side effects of glucagon may then be produced.

ADVANTAGES

Other than for insulinoma and phaeochromocytoma patients there are no real contra-indications when used for barium examinations. The paucity of side effects and their relatively minor character make glucagon, at the moment, the first choice in pharmacoradiology when myorelaxant is required, bearing in mind that it has no effect on oesophageal peristalsis.

SUMMARY AND CONCLUSIONS

The case for using pharmacoradiology has been argued previously[5] and is now largely accepted. Glucagon has, at present, a unique place in diagnostic radiology as a spasmolytic because of its widespread action on the stomach, duodenum, small bowel and colon and because of the low incidence of side effects and their relatively minor nature. With the increasing use of double contrast barium examinations, radiologists have become the largest users of this drug. With its relatively high cost, glucagon should be used at its lowest effective dose and then the price per injection compares favourably with other myorelaxants. It is also proving particularly valuable in computed tomography with devices having a scanning time of 18–20 seconds. Other uses include examination of post-operative and entero-biliary anastamoses, and in angiography, hystero-salpingography and possibly in excretion pyelography to show the ureters.

References

1   Meeroff, J. C., Jorgens, J. and Isenberg, J. I. (1975). The effect of glucagon on barium enema examination. *Radiology*, **115,** 5.

2   Unger, R. H. (1975). Action of glucagon as adjunct to gastrointestinal X-ray film examination. *J. Am. Med. Assoc.*, **231,** 80.

3   Lin, T. M. (1975). Actions of gastrointestinal hormones and related peptides on the motor function of biliary tract. *Gastroenterology*, **69,** 1006.

4   Rey, J. F. and Harvey, R. F. (1977). Hormonal control of the sphincter of Oddi. In J. Delmont, (ed.). *The Sphincter of Oddi*. Proceedings, 3rd Gastro-enterology Symp., Nice, 1976. pp. 66–71. (Basel: Karger)

5   Kreel, L. (1975). Pharmaco-radiology in barium examinations with special reference to glucagon. *Br. J. Radiol.*, **48,** 691.

6   Miller, R. E., Chernish, S. M., Brunelle, R. L. and Rosenak, B. D. (1978). Dose response to intramuscular glucagon during hypotonic radiography. *Radiology*, **127, 49.**

7   Miller, R. E., Chernish, S. M., Rosenak, B. D. and Rodda, B. E. (1973). Hypotonic duodenography with glucagon. *Radiology*, **108,** 35.

8   Miller, R. E., Chernish, S. M., Skucas, J., Rosenak, B. D. and Rodda, B. E. (1974). Hypotonic roentgenography with glucagon. *Am. J. Roentgenol.*, **121,** 264.

9   Miller, R. E., Chernish, S. M., Skucas, J., Rosenak, B. D. and Rodda, B. E. (1974). Hypotonic colon examination with glucagon. *Radiology*, **113,** 555.

10 Paul, F., Misaki, F. and Seifert, E. (1973). Crystalline pancreatic glucagon – a new spasmolytic agent: results of comparative endoscopic and electromanometric investigations in the proximal gastrointestinal tract. *Endoscopy*, **5,** 199.

11 Paul, F. and Freyschmidt, J. (1976). Anwendung von glukagon bei endo-skopischen und röntgenologischen Untersuchungen des Gastrointestinalt-rakts. *Fortschr. Röntgenstr.*, **125, 31.**

12 Barber, S. G. and Hamer, J. D. (1976). Skin rash in a patient receiving glucagon. *Lancet*, **ii,** 1138.

13 Kitabachi, A. E., Lamkin, N. Jr., Lieberman, P., Ayyagari, V. and Baskin, F. K. (1975). Allergic response to glucagon injection as a result of insulin contamination. *J. Clin. Endocrinol. Metab.*, **41,** 863.

14 Dalinka, M. K., Smith, E. H., Wolfe, R. D., Goldenberg, D. and Lorgdor, M. D. (1972). Pharmacologically enhanced visualization of oesophageal varices by pro-banthine. *Radiology*, **102,** 281.

15 Gohel, V. K., Dalinka, M. K. and Mandell, G. A. (1974). Pharma-coradiology of the gastrointestinal tract. *Crit. Rev. Clin. Radiol. Nucl. Med.*, **5** (1), 69.

16 Ghahremani, G. G., Heck, L. L. and Williams, J. R. (1972). A pharmacologic aid in the radiographic diagnosis of obstructive oesophageal lesions. *Radiology*, **103,** 289.

17 Cockerill, E. M., Miller, R. E., Chernish, S. M., McLaughlin III, G. C. and Rodda, B. E. (1976). Optimal visualization of esophageal varices. *Am. J. Roentgenol.*, **126** (3), 512.

18 Jennewein, H. M., Waldeck, F., Prahl, K. and Siewert, R. (1973). Zur Beeinflussung es unteren Osophagusspinkters durch gastrointestinale Hormone beim Hund. In R. Ottenjann, (ed.). *Refluxkrankheit der Speiserohre.* (Baden-Baden: Witzstrock).

19 Siewert, R., Fruh, E., Waldeck, F. *et al.* (1973). Senkung des Druckes im unteren Osophagusspinkter bei der Achalasie durch Glucagon. *Dtsch. Med., Worchenschr.*, **98,** 2045.

20 Ferrucci, J. T. Jr., and Long, J. A. (1977). Radiologic treatment of esophageal food impaction using intravenous glucagon. *Radiology*, **125,** 25.

21 Shirakabe, H. (1971). *Double Contrast Studies of the Stomach.* (Tokyo: Bunkodo).

22 Shirakabe, H., Ischikawa, H., Kumakura, K., Nishizawa, M., Higurashi, K., Hayakwa, H. and Murakami, T. (1972). *Atlas of Early X-ray Diagnosis of Early Gastric Cancer.* (Stuttgart: Thieme).

23 Dreiling, D. A. and Janowitz, H. D. (1959). The effect of glucagon on gastric secretion in man. *Gastroenterology*, **36,** 580.

24 op den Orth, O. O. and Ploem, S. (1977). The standard biphasic-contrast gastric series. *Radiology*, **122,** 530.

25 Liotta, D. (1955). Pour le diagnostic des tumeurs du pancreas: la duodeno-graphie hypertonique. *Lyon Chir.*, **50,** 445.

26 Jacquemet, P., Liotta, D. and Mallet-Guy, P. (1965). *The Early Radiological Diagnosis of Diseases of the Pancreas and Ampulla of Vater.* (Springfield: Charles C. Thomas).

27 Raia, S. and Kreel, L. (1966). Double contract gas distension duodenography using the Scott–Harden gastro-duodenal tube. *Gut*, **7,** 420.

28 Martel, W. (1968). Hypotonic duodenography without intubation. *Radiology*, **91,** 387.

29 Kreel, L. (1969). Duodenography in pancreatic disease with special reference to 'instant duodenography'. *Proc. R. Soc. Med.*, **62,** 881.

30 Kreel, L., Herlinger, H. and Glanville, J. (1973). Technique of the double contrast barium meal with examples of correlation with endoscopy. *Clin. Radiol.*, **24**, 307.

31 Chernish, S. M., Miller, R. E., Rosenak, B. D. and Scholz, N. E. (1972). Hypotonic duodenography with the use of glucagon. *Gastroenterology*, **63** (3), 392.

32 Jones, R. S. and Hall, A. D. (1969). The effect of glucagon on Brunner's gland secretion in dogs. *Proc. Soc. Exp. Biol. Med.*, **132**, 1159.

33 Gold, R. P. and Seaman, W. B. (1977). The primary double-contrast examination of the post-operative stomach. *Radiology*, **124**, 297.

34 Bilbao, M. K. and Dotter, C. T. (1975). Reflux cholangiography in sphincteroplasty or enterobiliary anastomosis. *Radiology*, **115**, 585.

35 Ferrucci, J. R. Jr., Wittenberg, J., Stone, L. B. and Dreyfuss, J. R. (1976). Hypotonic cholangiography with glucagon. *Radiology*, **118** (1), 466.

36 Dyck, W. P. and Janowitz, H. D. (1971). Effect of glucagon on hepatic bile secretion in man. *Gastroenterology*, **60**, 400.

37 Chernish, S. M., Miller, R. E., Rosenak, B. D. and Scholz, N. E. (1972). Effect of glucagon on size of visialized human gallbladder before and after a fat meal. *Gastroenterology*, **62**, 1218.

38 Kreel, L. (1975). The surface pattern of the stomach. *Proc. Soc. Med.*, **68** (2), 111.

39 Welin, S. (1958). Modern trends in diagnostic roentgenology of the colon. *Br. J. Radiol.*, **31**, 453.

40 Welin, S. (1967). Results of the Malmö technique of colon examination. *J. Am. Med. Assoc.*, **199**, 369.

41 Gohel, V. K., Dalinka, M. K. and Coren, G. S. (1975). Hypotonic examination of the colon with glucagon. *Radiology*, **115**, 1.

42 Taylor, I., Duthie, H. L., Cumberland, D. C. and Smallwood, R. (1975). Glucagon and the colon. *Gut*, **16**, 973.

43 Jerele, J. J. (1976). Use of glucagon as the hyptonic agent in barium enema examination. *J. Am. Osteopath. Assoc. (Chicago)*, **76**, 264.

44 Fisher, J. K. and Germann, D. R. (1977). Glucagon-aided reduction of intussusception. *Radiology*, **122**, 197.

45 Poser, H. and Baier, J. (1977). Vergleichende pharmako-dynamische Kolon-Doppelkontrastuntersuchung mit Glukagon und Atropin. *Radiol. Diagnostica*, **18**, 355.

46 Hradsky, M. and Furugard, K. (1976). Electrosurgical gastric polypectomy and duodenoscopy with the use of glucagon–Novo. *Scand. J. Gastroenterol.*, ·**11** (suppl. 38), 54.

47 Hradsky, M., Stockbrugger, R., Dotevall, G. and Ostberg, H. (1974). The use of glucagon during upper gastrointestinal endoscopy. *Gastrointest. Endosc.*, **20** (4), 162.

48 Madsen, J. E. Jr., Bonne, W. T., and Livstone, E. M. (1976). Endoscopic removal of a dental instrument from the stomach. *Am. J. Gastroenterol.*, **66** (4), 377.

49 Cotton, P. B. (1972). Progress report: cannulation of the Papilla of Vater by endoscopy and retrograde cholangiopancreatography (ERCP). *Gut,* **13,** 1004.

50 Katon, R. M., Lee, T. G., Parent, J. A., Bilbao, M. K. and Smith, F. W. (1974). Endoscopic retrograde cholangiopancreatography (ERCP). Experience with 100 cases. *Am. J. Digest Dis.,* **19,** 295.

51 Schmidt, F. W. (1973). Crystalline pancreatic glucagon – a new spasmodic agent: results of comparative endoscopic and electromanometric investigations in the proximal gastrointestinal tract. *Endoscopy,* **5,** 199.

52 Koch, H., Belohlavek, D., Schaffner, O., Tympner, F., Rosch, W. and Demling, L. (1975). Prospective study for the prevention of pancreatitis following endoscopic retrograde cholangiopancreatography (ERCP). *Endoscopy,* **7,** 221.

53 Silvis, S. E. and Vennes, J. A. (1975). The role of glucagon in endoscopic cholangiopancreatography. *Gastrointest. Endosc.,* **21,** 162.

54 Kreel, L. (1970). Menstrual irregularities and infertility. *Radiology,* **6,** 887.

55 Gerlock, A. J. and Hooser, C. W. (1976). Oviduct response to glucagon during hysterosalpingography. *Radiology,* **119,** 727.

56 Shoemaker, W. C., van Italie, T. B. and Walker, W. F. (1959). Measurement of hepatic glucose output and hepatic blood flow in response to glucagon. *Am. J. Physiol.,* **196,** 315.

57 Merrill, S. L., Chvojka, V. E., Berkowitz, G. M. and Texter, E.C. Jr. (1962). Effects of glucagon on superior mesenteric vascular bed. *Fed. Proc.,* **21,** 200.

58 Danford, R. O. and Davidson, A. J. (1969). The use of glucagon as a vasodilater in visceral angiography. *Radiology,* **93** (1), 173.

59 Danford, R. O. (1970). The effect of glucagon on renal hemodynamics and renal arteriography. *Am. J. Roentgenol.,* **108** (4), 665.

60 Lowman, R. M., Belleza, N. A., Goetsch, J. B., Finkelstein, H. I., Berneike, R. R. and Rosenfield, A. T. (1977). Glucagon. *J. Urol.,* **118,** 128.

61 Lefebvre, J. and Unger, R. H. (eds.). (1972). *Glucagon,* p. 370. (Oxford: Pergamon).

62 Kreel, L. (1976). The EMI Whole Body Scanner: An interim clinical evaluation of the prototype. *Br. J. Clin. Equip.,* **4,** 1016.

63 Paul, F. (1978). Personal communication.

DISCUSSION

Jaspan: I would like to try to answer some of your questions about the physiological side effects of glucagon. Although provocative tests to stimulate release of catecholamines, e.g. histamine, tyramine, and glucagon, were popular in the late 60s and early 70s, with the advent of more sophisticated and accurate biochemical tests for catecholamines and their metabolites in plasma and urine, the current trend is away from the use of these agents. This is because (i) they can be dangerous, and occasionally even lethal, and, short of actual danger, are frequently associated with very unpleasant side effects, (ii) they *all* carry false positives and false negatives, and (iii) they seldom offer anything more than the conventional biochemical tests available today. Thus their use today is restricted by most endocrinologists (including myself and those with whom I work) to the very unusual case in which such a diagnosis is strongly suspected, but in which all conventional tests are negative. In these rare circumstances the advantages of histamine, tyramine, glucagon, or tilting procedures are still disputed, each having its proponents and opponents. In general, this is the theme running throughout recent literature in this area. Key references include: Anton, A.H. and Goldberg, L.I. (1974), in *The Heart* (J. Willis Hurst and R. Bruce Logue, eds.) pp. 1212–1223; Remine, W.H. *et al.* (1974), *Ann. Surg.*, **179**, 740; Editorial (1967), *N. Engl. J. Med.*, **227**, 762; White *et al.* (1973), *Res. Comm. Chem. Path. Pharm.*, **5**, 252.

Kreel: Is it true that phaeochromocytoma is an absolute contraindication to using glucagon? I would add that I have issued instructions in my department that in no circumstances is glucagon to be used in insulinomas or in phaeochromocytomas. In order to be quite clear, from your study of the literature, Dr Jaspan, what doses have been found to be dangerous?

Jaspan: The usual doses that have been used in provocative tests are, I believe, 1 mg or 2 mg intravenously.

Kreel: In my opinion, this drug is otherwise perfectly safe. It has been used in cardiology for many years. It is also carried by many diabetics for hypoglycaemia. If there is a hypersensitivity, could it be that this is due to insulin contamination?

Jaspan: That is a possibility, but that would only be encountered in diabetics on injections of less purified forms of insulin (such as some of those available in the USA). Incidentally, I share your concern about the term 'spasmolytic', which implies a pathologic or pathogenic entity. Perhaps 'hypotonic' or 'atonic' would be a better word.

Kreel: I thought about 'hypotonic' for a long time, but that really refers to osmolality. What is needed is a word that describes the 'relaxing' properties of these agents.

Myren: Personally, I am reluctant to use sedatives and anti-cholinergics in out-patients, and about 50% of our endoscopies are performed on such people. To move to another point, we, and others, have often found a poor correlation between symptoms and what the radiologist finds in the digestive tract. I would like to ask Dr Kreel if he was using glucagon in the double contrast studies he has done, and if he found this helpful as far as accurate diagnosis was concerned.

Kreel: Yes, glucagon was used in the cases I was talking about. In my opinion, if one does not do a double contrast examination one misses a number of lesions. Using this technique, with either glucagon or hyoscine butyl bromide, it is possible to demonstrate lesions which would not otherwise be found. Small ulcer scars, chronic erosive gastritis, and polyps in the stomach, for instance, are now routinely being diagnosed, which was not the case before we had this technique. We have, incidentally, done a very carefully controlled comparative test between endoscopy and radiology, and found radiology almost to match endoscopy as far as diagnosis is concerned.

Paul: I have found glucagon to be a very useful agent in the diagnosis of abnormalities of the biliary tree. Radiologists often refer patients to me with the suggestion that I perform an endoscopic sphincterotomy, thinking that the patient complaining of abdominal pain and showing pre-papillary narrowing of a slightly 'dilated' common bile duct might· have papillary stenosis or sclerosis. In my experience this X-ray diagnosis is nearly always wrong. The administration of glucagon and a repeat of the radiological examination usually clarifies the situation, and shows an endoscopic sphincterotomy to be unnecessary. As far as side effects of glucagon are concerned, I recall once having induced a hypertensive crisis in a case of phaeochromocytoma. Admittedly, such patients are not often seen, but since then we have always been careful not to administer this substance to them. Some people are certainly more sensitive than others to glucagon. A rare patient may vomit after a dose of only 0.3 mg, for instance, whereas most will tolerate two to four times that dose with no side effects. I do not know why this is. It obviously is not weight-dependent. One can always continue the infusion after lowering the dose of the hormone.

Wingate: To my mind, one of the problems when studying the digestive tract, is that of terminology. It seems to me that we do not all mean exactly the same thing when we talk of 'motility', 'transit', 'pressure', and so on. As a result, to some extent at least, we are all measuring different things, in different ways, and then drawing impermissible conclusions about what is happening. The more work we all do, the more extensive our terminology, and so the more confusing the whole matter becomes. It seems to be that a lot of things would become more clear if this matter of terminology could be straightened out.

Kreel: Yes indeed.

6 Biliary Surgery, Radiomano-metry and Glucagon

M.-J. Treffot, F. Quilichini and M.-F. Vinson

Disturbances occurring during bile duct emptying may be due either to an anomaly of motoricity or to an organic lesion of the sphincter of Oddi. These disturbances can be detected and differentiated by means of surgical radiomanometry, and upon the findings a decision can be made regarding further surgery.

In the anaesthetized subject the motoricity of the biliary tract is always modified by drugs; the competitive neuro-muscular blocking agents act as muscle relaxants, while neuro-leptics and morphine (or morphine derivatives) cause muscular contractions.[1] During surgical radiomanometry it is therefore necessary to use drugs which act on the choledochal sphincter, but whose effects do not mask any spasmodic or organic abnormalities. Amyl nitrite is usually used for this purpose. This substance, however, is not without disadvantages both for the patient and for the anaesthetist.[2] Glucagon was considered as an alternative as the myorelaxant effects of this substance on the stomach, duodenum,[3] and colon were known, and its use during the radiological study of the bile duct, [4][5] and to antagonize the effects of morphinics during surgical radiomanometry, has already been proposed.[6][7] The present study was designed to test its value as a myorelaxant on the biliary tract during surgical radiomanometry, and to see if it would permit a distinction to be made between the spasmodic and the organic abnormalities.

MATERIAL AND METHODS

Surgical radiomanometry was carried out in 21 patients, ten male and eleven female, whose ages ranged from 29 to 78. Surgery was performed in emergency situations in six instances,

TABLE 6.1 Effect of glucagon on 21 patients subjected to surgical radiomanometry

Patient number	Age	Sex	Diagnosis	Emergency	Bile duct lesions[a]	Gallbladder lesions	Glucagon dose (µg/kg)	Radiological effect	Emptying effect[c]	Resting pressure[b] before glucagon	Resting pressure[b] after glucagon
1	69	M	Pyocholecyst	++	0	Lithiasis; pus	4	++	++	–	9
2	48	F	Biliary colic	–	0	Lithiasis	10	+++	++	–	8
3	69	F	Cholangitis	–	Lithiasis (+)	Lithiasis	4	+	+	11	8
4	46	M	Chronic pancreatitis	–	(+)	0	4	+	++(*)	12	9
5	43	M	Acute pancreatitis	+	0	0	10	+	++(*)	25	20
6	65	F	Biliary colic	–	0	Lithiasis	4	++	+	10	8
7	32	F	Acute pancreatitis	++	(+)	Lithiasis	4	++	++(*)	12	9
8	67	M	Biliary colic	–	0	Lithiasis	10	++	+++(*)	13	10
9	55	M	Icterus	–	(+)	Lithiasis	4	+++	+	11	9.5
10	29	F	Biliary colic	–	0	Lithiasis	4	+	++	11	8
11	67	F	Biliary colic	+	(+)	Lithiasis	10	+++	++	20	10
12	73	M	Icterus	+	(+)	Lithiasis	10	++++	+++(*)	18	15
13	33	F	Biliary colic	+	(+)	Cholecystitis	10	++	+++(*)	10	8
14	70	M	Cholecystitis	–	0	Cholecystitis	10	++	+	12	9
15	68	M	Biliary colic	–	0	Atrophy	10	0	0(*)	25	25
16	44	F	Biliary colic	–	0	Lithiasis	4	0	0(*)	25	25
17	77	M	Cholangitis	–	(+)	Atrophy	4	0	0	10	10
18	73	M	Biliary colic	–	Lithiasis (+)	Lithiasis	4	0	0(*)	16	16
19	78	F	Biliary colic	–	(+)	Atrophy / Lithiasis	AN¶ / 4	0	0(*)	16	16
20	65	F	Pyocholecyst	+	Lithiasis (+)	Atrophy / Lithiasis	AN¶ / 4	0	0(*)	18	15
21	78	F	Biliary colic	–	0	Lithiasis	AN¶ / 4	0	0(*)	10	10

[a]Bile duct lesions: (+) = dilatation
¶AN = 0.3 ml amyl nitrite inhaled

[b]Resting pressure is expressed in cmH$_2$O

[c]Emptying effect: (*) = emptying obtained only with glucagon

four for cholecystitis and two for acute pancreatitis. In ten of the other cases it was performed for non-complicated gallbladder lithiasis, in four for complicated gallbladder lithiasis, and in one for pancreas associated diseases (see Table 6.1). Droperidol 10–20 mg/kg and atropine 0.25 mg were used as premedication, and anaesthesia was induced with thiopenthal 6–8 mg/kg and suxamethonium chloride 1 mg/kg. Neuroleptanalgesia was maintained with Fentanyl 0.5 mg and droperidol 30–40 mg, and relaxation was obtained with pancuronium bromide 4–6 mg.

Radiomanometry was carried out in the classical way after the insertion of a cannula into the cystic duct. The contrast medium used was Vasobrix 32. The filling of the bile duct with the contrast medium was viewed on a fluoroscopic screen, and radiographs were taken at the following stages: (a) during the filling of the bile duct, under low pressure, (b) during the filling of the common duct and of the right and left hepatic ducts, under increased pressure, and (c) whilst emptying through the sphincter of Oddi. Three pressure levels were recorded: full filling pressure (FP), emptying pressure (EP), and resting or residual pressure (RP). The effects of glucagon studied were those on the dynamic fluoroscopic aspects, the bile duct emptying phase, the EP and RP, and the cardiovascular system.

Glucagon was administered intravenously, and the dose was 4 μg/kg for twelve patients, and 10 μg/kg for the other nine. Amyl nitrite 0.3 ml was administered to four of the patients in whom glucagon was ineffective (see below) and these patients were then re-subjected to the radiological and pressure recording procedures described above.

RESULTS

Glucagon was seen to be effective in 14 of the 21 patients. The radiological findings show there to be three distinct stages of activity. Firstly, there is a short phase of paradoxical contraction, clearly seen on the fluoroscopic screen, which starts within one minute and which lasts for less than one minute. Secondly, there is a phase of relaxation, which is quickly followed, thirdly, by an increase in the emptying of bile duct contents into the duodenum. The effect disappears within five minutes.

The EP is reduced. In six patients, in fact, the emptying of the bile duct was only obtained after the administration of glucagon (Table 6.1). The RP was significantly reduced in 12 of the 14 patients in whom glucagon was effective. In seven patients no emptying occurred. In one of these patients, however, a fall in the RP was seen after the administration of 0.4 mg glucagon.

No undesirable side effects were seen in any of the 21 patients. It is especially worth noting that no changes occurred in the arterial pressure nor in the pulse rate. .

DISCUSSION

The idea that gut hormones might be involved in the control of the motility of the biliary tract led to the extraction of cholecystokinin from the duodenal wall by Ivy and Oldberg in 1928.[8] The effects of glucagon have been known for only ten years. Excluding the metabolic effects, the main property of this hormone is a myorelaxant activity. The effect appears in the stomach, duodenum, small intestine and colon, and glucagon is used during radiological explorations of these organs and during endoscopic investigations.[9-11]

The myorelaxant effect of glucagon is seen in the whole of the biliary tract. In the conscious dog the effect on the gallbladder is dose-dependent, and appears after doses as low as $0.25 \mu g/kg$.[12 13] In man glucagon produces a significant increase in the size of the gallbladder,[10] but this effect has not been shown *in vitro*.[14] Lin has observed a biphasic effect at the bile duct level in the conscious cat: the decrease of choledochal resistance being occasionally preceded by an increase in pressure after doses of $5 \mu g/kg$ or more.[15] This biphasic effect was seen in the present study.

This effect on the muscle results in a fall in the intracholedochal pressure during filling and emptying, and in the resting pressure. This phenomenon was noted in the present study: emptying occurred at lower pressures after the administration of glucagon than before. In six patients emptying was obtained only after the administration of glucagon.

The resting pressure was seen to fall significantly amongst

TABLE 6.2 Effect of glucagon on resting pressure

	Effective *(12 patients)*	*Non-effective* *(7 patients)*
Before glucagon	13.8 ± 4	17.8 ± 5.7
After glucagon	10 ± 3.4	17.8 ± 5.7
	$(p < 0.0005)$	

Pressure expressed in cmH_2O

the twelve patients tested before and after glucagon administration. The mechanism of this action is not clear. The relaxation occurs in all muscles involved in maintaining the sphincter tone and the intra-choledochal pressure, i.e. the gallbladder and bile duct muscles, and those of the duodenal wall.[16] It may be that glucagon works directly on the sphincter[17-19]; it may also be that a decrease in the bile output enhances the muscular effects.[20-22] If one regards as physiological the hormone levels necessary to act on carbohydrate metabolism, it seems that the doses of hormone required for such an action are super-physiological or pharmacological.

The myorelaxant effect of glucagon appears to be similar to that of amyl nitrite. Certainly, when one substance failed to have an effect in the present study, the second was similarly ineffective. It is notable, incidentally, that the four patients in whom this occurred were among the oldest studied, and that in all four instances the gallbladder was found to be atrophic.

Surgical exploration in all 21 patients confirmed the accuracy of the radiomanometric findings, i.e. in all seven patients in whom glucagon proved ineffective, thereby suggesting an organic lesion of the sphincter of Oddi, this was indeed found to be the case, whilst in the fourteen patients in whom glucagon was effective the normality of the sphincter was confirmed.

CONCLUSION

In conclusion it may be said that whilst glucagon and amyl nitrite appear to be equally good myorelaxants of the biliary tract, the ease of use and lack of undesirable side effects of glucagon make this the preferred substance, certainly during surgical radiomanometry.

References

1 Kantor, E., Jakab, T. and Szabo, L. (1969). Der einfluss der neuroleptanalgesic auf dein tonus der sphincter der Oddi. *Anaesthetist*, **18**, 183.

2 Vinson, M.-F., Treffot, M.-J. and Quilichini, F. (1977). Radiomanométrie biliaire: intérêt du glucagon. *N. Presse Med.*, **6**, 2897.

3 Miller, R. E., Chernish, S. M., Rosenak, B. D. and Rodda, B. E. (1973). Hypotonic duodenography with glucagon. *Radiology*, **108**, 35.

4 Bilbao, M. K. and Dotter, C. T. (1975). Reflux cholangiography in sphincteroplasty or enterobiliary anastomosis. *Radiology*, **115**, 585.

5 Ferrucci, J. T., Wittenberg, J., Stone, L. B. and Dreyfuss, J. R. (1976). Hypotonic cholangiography with glucagon. *Radiology*, **118**, 466.

6 Neidhardt, A., Garrigues, M., Neidhardt-Audion, M., Kobi-Kabbas, F. and Hamdouch, A. (1977). Analgésie et voies biliaries. Compatibilité parfaite et méconnue. *Anesth. Anal. Réan.*, **34**, 901.

7 Pire, J. C., Burde, A., Flament, J. B. and Rives, J. (1976). Utilisation des morphinomimétiques en chirurgie biliaire. *N. Presse Med.*, **5**, 1838.

8 Ivy, A. C. and Oldberg, E. (1928). A hormonal mechanism for gallbladder contraction and evacuation. *Am. J. Physiol.*, **86**, 599.

9 von Brandstatter, G. and Kratochvil, P. (1977). Anwendungsmöglichkeiten von Glukagon im bereich der gastrointestinalen endoskopie. *Arch. Arzneitherapie*, **1**, 172.

10 Chernish, S. M., Miller, R. E., Rosenak, B. D. and Scholz, N. E. (1972). Hypotonic duodenography with the use of glucagon. *Gastroenterology*, **63**, 392.

11 Paul, F., Misaki, F. and Seifert, E. (1973). Crystalline pancreatic glucagon – a new spasmolytic agent: results of comparative endoscopic and electromanometric investigations in the proximal gastrointestinal tract. *Endoscopy*, **5**, 199.

12 Lin, T. M. (1971). Hepatic, cholecystokinetic and choledochal actions of natural gastrointestinal polypeptides. *Post Graduate Course, Am. Gastroenterol. Assoc.*

13 Lin, T. M. (1974). Action of secretin, glucagon, cholecystokinin and endogenously released secretin and cholecystokinin on gallbladder, choledochus and bile flow in dogs. *Fed. Proc.*, **33**, 391.

14 Cameron, A. J., Phillips, S. F. and Summerskill, W. H. J. (1969). Effect of

cholecystokinin, gastrin, secretin and glucagon on human gallbladder muscle *in vitro*. *Proc. Soc. Exp. Biol. Med.,* **131,** 149.

15   Lin, T. M. (1975). Actions of gastrointestinal hormones and related peptides on the motor function of the biliary tract. *Gastroenterology,* **69,** 1006.

16   Audigier, J. C., Vatne, M., Fargier, M. C. and Decultieux, A. (1972). Effet cholécystokinétique des hormones gastrointestinales. *Biol. Gastroentérol. (Paris),* **5,** 287.

17   Andersson, K. E., Andersson, R., Hedner, P. and Persson, C. G. A. (1972). Effect of cholecystokinin on the level of cyclic AMP and on mechanical activity in the isolated sphincter of Oddi. *Life Sci.,* **11,** 723.

18   Nagee, D. F. (1946). Some observations on the pharmacology of the sphincter of Oddi. *J. Pharm. Pharmacol.,* **19,** 38.

19   Rey, J. F. and Harvey, R. F. (1977). Hormonal control of the sphincter of Oddi. In J. Delmont, (ed.). *The sphincter of Oddi.* Proceedings, 3rd Gastroenterology Symp., Nice, 1976. pp. 66–71. (Basel: Karger).

20   Chernish, S. M., Miller, R. E., Rosenak, B. D. and Scholz, N. E. (1972). Effect of glucagon on size of visualized human gallbladder before and after a fat meal. *Gastroenterology,* **62,** 1218.

21   Dyck, W. P. and Janowitz, H. D. (1971). Effect of glucagon on hepatic bile secretion in man. *Gastroenterology,* **60,** 400.

22   Lin, T. M. and Spray, G. F. (1969). Effect of pentagastrin, cholecystokinin, caerulein and glucagon on the choledochal resistance and bile flow in the dog. *Gastroenterology,* **56,** 1178.

7 Biliary Radiomanometry as an Investigative Tool in Biliary Tract Disease

J. D. McCarthy

Of what use would it be to know the minimum pressure in the bile duct existant at the moment of flow through the sphincter of Oddi? Does the number describing the pressure give us information we can apply? Do the numbers derived add to our understanding of disease processes? Do effective therapeutic decisions follow? And, for the sake of this workshop, is radiomanometry a useful method by which we can better understand the use of glucagon on the biliary tree?

We can reason by analogy and point out the spectacular progress of cardiology based upon quantitation of pressures and flow or the new insights into the understanding of oesophageal reflux or into diverticular disease of the colon. But, although these and other modalities are well accepted, biliary radiomanometry is still little used, especially in the United States. A moment's reflection upon that fact may be appropriate.

Since biliary operations are among the most frequently performed, e.g. 500000 cholecystectomies annually in the United States, each of a great number of surgeons may pose as an expert on the basis of his own experience. It is also true that biliary tract operations are among the safest and most satisfactory major operations and thus recognized defects in the performance of the operation are soon forgotten, the lesson being erased by good results. Awareness of unrecognized defects is even more remote. These in turn lead to a sense of satisfaction in one's own competence. Understandable scepticism nurtures a reasonable reluctance not to incorporate every new suggestion into practice, so that even such a clearly useful technique as syringe injection per-operative cholangiography is not routine for many. Then, after all that, the special apparatus and new concepts promote a final reluctance. I believe radiomanometry is used widely by European surgeons, but I do not know specifically how widely.

APPARATUS AND TECHNIQUE

A simple U manometer (Figure 7.1) is the basic unit of the

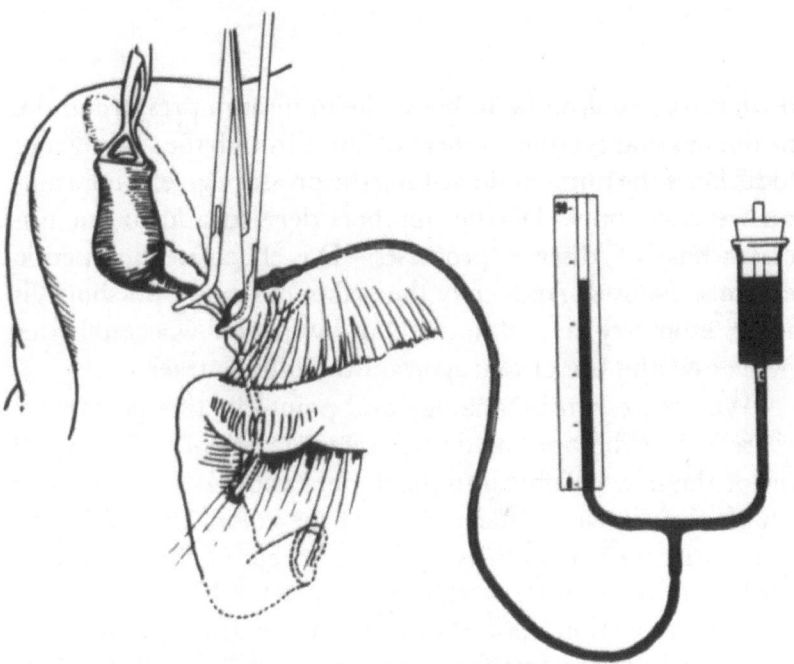

Figure 7.1 Representation of manometer and its attachment to the cannula which has been inserted into the common bile duct via the cystic duct. The zero point is the level of the sphincter of Oddi

system. The liquid in the calibrated arm reflects the pressure surrounding the cannula in the common bile duct. The system is inelegant, has the inertia of a fluid system, but fortunately is inexpensive, easily sterilized and simple to use. As flow out of the system takes place, entry of air to replace the fluid is easily gauged by watching for air motion in the glass tube perforating the stopper in the reservoir. The contrast fluid filling the whole system is diatrizoate sodium 50% (Hypaque) diluted in equal portion with saline. A metallic cannula (Champeau) is passed through the cystic duct into the choledochus. The zero level of the manometer is adjusted so as to correspond to the level of the sphincter of Oddi and the height of the reservoir which controls the pressure of the system dropped to a low level. All valves are opened and the reservoir (pressure) elevated gradually until evidence of beginning flow is seen. Radiographs are taken to assure that the flow through the sphincter has taken place (a dilated biliary tree can appear to be a normal conduit), and that there are no concretions in the biliary tree.

REPRODUCIBILITY

Hess,[1] Albot *et al.*,[2] Mallet-Guy[3] and Yvergneaux[4] have suggested that the upper limit of normal pressure to bypass the sphincter of Oddi, that is, passage pressure, is 15 cmH$_2$O or less. We too have used this number as the upper limits of normal, and have found it meaningful.[5] It seems to incorporate at least 90% of some 300 normal studies. Daniel,[6] White[7] and Mieny[8] indicate that the upper limit of normal passage pressure may be somewhat higher, up to 18 cmH$_2$O. The zone 15 to 20 cmH$_2$O pressure is admittedly a difficult area through which to judge potentiality for significant choledochal disease. A 2 cm error in zero levelling is not unreasonable although probably infrequent. A 1 cm error in specifying passage pressure is also not unreasonable. Thus, a few centimetres of abnormal elevation in passage pressure might be normal although we[9] and others have found small choledocholiths in patients in that range.

Concern about the possible spasmogenic effect of the infused contrast material, although reasonable, has been allayed by direct investigations. Neither Cushieri *et al.*[10] nor Hess,[1] p. 248, could measure such an effect at the customary dilutions of the contrast liquid.

Further supporting the reproducibility of the method is that the operator can return repeatedly to confirm the level of the passage pressure.[11] That so many authors have suggested approximately the same range of normal pressure and that these correspond to our own confirms that the same phenomenon is being measured and that systematic errors are not nullifying.

Control of the adequacy of the determination of the passage pressure is the determination of the resting or residual pressure. When the tube to the manometer's reservoir is clamped, fluid flows from the calibrated column until it equilibrates with the residual pressure of the choledochus, which when normal is invariably less than the passage pressure, usually 2 to 4 cmH$_2$O less. If this relation does not exist, then a technical defect or organic obstruction to flow should be considered. If passage pressure is normal and the roentgenogram does not indicate any abnormality, I often omit determination of the resting pressure. In brief, this technique is reproducible, both in my operating room and across the world.

Does the information from radiomanometry add to the understanding of disease processes? Consider the problem of jaundice in an obese patient undergoing an operation because of acute cholecystitis. Does the jaundice represent choledocholithiasis and thereby a difficult and possibly dangerous common duct exploration, or does it represent cholestasis or ascending pericholangitis or transcholecystic escape of bile? A cholecystectomy followed by a normal radiomanometric study will remove any necessity to explore the common duct. I have personally seen this at least six times. Further, if the study is abnormal, the surgeon has a lighter heart about extending the operation.

In a recent study of 198 patients who had radiomanometry, I identified fourteen patients with cholecystolithiasis who, although they had no history of jaundice or pancreatitis and had normal serum bilirubin and alkaline phosphatase levels, displayed elevated passage pressures. Nine of these seemingly normal patients had choledocholithiasis. Only two patients were normal and three probably had papillitis.[9]

We recently performed a cholecystectomy and produced a radiomanometric study easily within the normal range on a 33-year-old woman. Following the operation, we were informed that pre-operatively she had an elevation of serum alkaline phosphatase to about three times normal. However, in view of the normal manometric studies, we dismissed the applicability of further operations or more complex diagnostic work, e.g.

endoscopic retrograde cholangio-pancreatography (ERCP). She rapidly recovered. Thus, the information from radiomanometry clearly bears upon the disease processes.

Do effective therapeutic decisions follow the information gained from radiomanometry? As suggested in the introduction, this question is harder to answer because the prudent surgeon, using operative cholangiography, but not using manometry, will but infrequently fall into error even though his understanding is less complete. In a study[9] I suggested that in 3.7% of biliary operations done in my area, choledocholithiasis is overlooked. However, the frequency of clinically retained or recurrent common bile duct calculi is nowhere near that percentage, implying that these smaller stones typically pass. Acosta and Ledesma displayed quite convincingly that surprisingly large stones may pass the sphincter.[11] It should be stated that radiomanometry may lead to common duct explorations to remove calculi that if left alone would spontaneously pass.

The abnormalities of the sphincter of Oddi and the papilla of Vater is a chapter still being written.[12] That inflammatory and fibrotic changes, probably post-inflammatory in origin, may be found by radiomanometry is indisputable, but their roles in symptomatology or in the pathogenesis of pancreatitis and cholelithiasis are not clear to me. I use elevated passage pressure and elevated resting pressures that are not due to an impacted calculus in the presence of a normal or small common bile duct as partial indication for sphincteroplasty.[13] I have, however, nagging doubts that operation is always necessary.

RADIOMANOMETRY AND GLUCAGON

Vinson, Treffot and Quilichini[14] recently reported that glucagon given during radiomanometric investigation of the choledochus resulted in a relaxation of the sphincter of Oddi. They pointed out that such a non-toxic agent as glucagon is much to be preferred over amyl nitrite with its complexity of administration and induced arterial hypotension. The mechanism of relaxation, that is the decrease in choledochal

TABLE 7.1 Effect of glucagon on sphincter of Oddi: measurements of residual pressure (RP) (determined after passage pressure (PP)) and volume infused during one minute at 30 cm H_2O pressure (White et al.[7]) (TF). All determinations done between 3 to 5 minutes following bolus IV injection of 1 mg glucagon

	Pre-glucagon			Post-glucagon			
Patient: sex: age	PP	RP	TF	PP	RP	TF	Diagnosis: remarks
FM:F:50	13	11	26	—	—	31	Cholecytolithiasis: normal CBD
DC:F:58	12	7	14	—	10	12	Cholecytolithiasis: normal CBD
IR:M:68	10	7	12	10	7	12	Acute cholecystitis: multiple calculi
DL:F:32	6	—	19	—	—	19	Chronic cholecystitis: possible hepatitis
MB:F:90	>30	>30	0	>30	>30	0	Jaundice, acalculous cholecystitis: primary stenosing papillitis. Choldocho-duodenostomy. Autopsy 6 weeks later.
AO:F:86	29	25	2	—	29	3	Chronic cholecystitis with lithiasis pancreatitis with abscess 6 years before. Recent suspect pancreatitis. Suspect papillitis secondary to duodenal diverticulum. Negative common duct exploration. T-tube placed.
BC:F:27	12	9.5	20	—	9.5	20	RUQ pain, 9 years after cholecystectomy ERCP suggested choledocholithiasis. Alkaline phosphatase 2.5 × normal. CBD not explored: radiographically normal at operation.
DV:F:58	18	—	1	omitted			Cholecysto- and choledocholithiasis: T-tube placed.
	15	10	—	15	10		5 days post-op: T-tube
NC:F:72	>50						Manometry: radiographs – Negative 1 yr post-cholecystojejunostomy for 'Ca of pancreas'. ERCP = choledocholithiasis. Cholecystectomy choledocholithotomy.
	21			17			T-tube 7 days post-op: T-tube manometry residual calculus. Start heparin irrigation 6 days later, normal cholangiogram. Manometry not done.

pressure, could not be specified, they explained, without examining the isolated sphincter of Oddi. Let us consider some propositions while thinking through their statements. First, duodenal relaxation rapidly follows intravenous glucagon. Second, compressive closure of the intramural portion of the common bile duct by duodenal contraction is easily relieved. Third, elevated intraluminal duodenal pressure may change the normal emptying pressure of the common bile duct. However the sphincter of Oddi seems to be an independent muscular unit and, as such, would be expected to perform oppositely from the duodenal wall musculature. Among patients so far tested personally (Table 7.1), no or only equivocal evidence of relaxation of the sphincter of Oddi by intravenous glucagon has been recorded. We tested the passage pressure, then residual pressure and then we followed White's[7] suggestion of a dynamic measurement of volume of flow through the sphincter for one minute at $30\,cm\,H_2O$ pressure. Residual pressure was again determined so as to be sure that spasm had not been induced by the elevated pressure. Then glucagon 1 mg was given intravenously. After a standardized wait of three minutes during which time the residual pressure was constantly measured, the passage pressure was redetermined as was volume flow (timed flow (TF) on Table 7.1) all within the next two minutes. Our radiological colleagues assure us that glucagon is effective during that period of time. Why this difference should exist is deeply interesting. Those authors gave $10\,\mu g/kg$ body weight. We gave all patients 1 mg or about $16{-}17\,\mu g/kg$. 1 mg is quite satisfactory for hypotonic duodenography for most patients.

SUMMARY

Radiomanometry is a useful modality for the investigation of biliary tract disease among humans during operative procedures. It is safe and accurate, and new and useful information comes from its employment. Information gathered through its use is contradictory as regards the effect of glucagon on the sphincter of Oddi.

References

1   Hess, W. (1965). *Surgery of the Biliary Passages and the Pancreas*. (New York: D. van Nostrand).
2   Albot, G., Olivier, C. and Libaude, H. (1953). Radiomanometric examination of the biliary ducts: experience with 418 cases. *Gastroenterology*, **24,** 242.
3   Mallet-Guy, P. (1952). Value of preoperative manometric and roentgenographic examinations in the diagnosis of functional disturbances of the biliary tract. *Surg. Gynecol. Obstet.*, **94,** 385.
4   Yvergneaux, J. P., Bauwens, E. and Yvergneaux, E. (1974). Diagnostic de la stenose Oddienne bénigne dans une série homogene de 1150 interventions biliares sous radiomanométrie. *Ann. Chir.*, **28,** 545.
5   McCarthy, J. D. (1970). Radiomanometry during biliary operations. *Arch. Surg.*, **100,** 424.
6   Daniel, O. (1972). Value of radiomanometry in bile duct surgery. *Ann. Roy. Coll. Surg. Engl.*, **51,** 357.
7   White, T. T., Waisman, H., Hoptom, D. and Kavlie, H. (1972). Radiomanometry, flow rates and cholangiography in the evaluation of common bile duct disease. *Am. J. Surg.*, **123,** 73.
8   Mieny, C. J.; Mendelow, D. and Cooke, M. B. (1974). Radiomanometry in the diagnosis of common bile duct disease. *S. Afr. J. Surg.*, **12,** 189.
9   McCarthy, J. D. (1977). Radiomanometric guides to common duct exploration. *Am. J. Surg.*, **134,** 697.
10 Cushieri, A., Hughes, J. H. and Cohen, M. (1972). Biliary pressure studies during cholecystectomy. *Br. J. Surg.*, **59,** 267.
11 Acosta, M. and Ledesma, C. L. (1974). Gallstone migration as a cause of acute pancreatitis. *N. Engl. J. Med.*, **290,** 484.
12 Delmont, J. (ed.). (1977). *The Sphincter of Oddi*. (Basel: Karger).
13 Jones, S. A., Steedman, R. A., Keller, T. B. and Smith, L. L. (1969). Transduodenal sphincteroplasty for biliary and pancreatic disease: indications, contraindications, and results. *Am. J. Surg.*, **118,** 292.
14 Vinson, M.-E., Treffot, M.-J. and Quilichini, F. (1977). Radiomanométrie biliare: intérêt du glucagon. *Nouv. Presse Med.*, **6,** 2897.

DISCUSSION

(Editor's note: Unfortunately, at the last minute Dr Treffot was unable to go to Madrid for this workshop. In her absence her paper was read to the participants by the chairman, and was not separately discussed. In the discussion which followed the presentation of Professor McCarthy's paper several points were raised which related to Dr Treffot's paper rather than to his, but it has been decided to include

these here, since there is, after all, a considerable overlap between the two authors fields of interest.)

Wingate: I would like to mention two physiological points at this stage. The first is that the group at Nottingham University which has been doing work similar to ours with dogs, has looked very closely at the effect of the bolus injection of glucagon. They have found that the initial effect of the bolus injection, which lasts between two and four minutes, is, in fact, an intense stimulation of intestinal activity, and that this is then superseded by a cessation of the myoelectric activity. One sees first the stimulation by glucagon, and then a catecholamine release from the paralysis of the whole system. This, I think, is the biphasic effect mentioned by Dr Treffot.

The second point is that Mr Hilary Thompson of the Department of Experimental Surgery at the London Hospital has recently done some studies in order to try to demonstrate the difference between the sphincter itself, in terms of muscle, and the duodenum. Although there is a separate muscle in the sphincter, it has apparently proved virtually impossible to get it to act independently of the duodenum. This also means that when the duodenum relaxes, the whole sphincter relaxes as well.

McCarthy: I would like to point out that if the sphincter of Oddi relaxes when the duodenum relaxes, as with hypotonic duodenography, one should see filling of the common bile duct upon external pressure.

Wingate: I think that would depend on the pressure within the biliary tree, for it is not only the sphincter which stops reflux.

Kreel: No, there is a sort of flap valve, and the more pressure put on this valve the more tightly it remains closed. The most interesting thing in all this, to my mind, is that when the whole system relaxes the contrast can flow backwards from the common bile duct into the duct of Wirsung. This suggests that there is a constant normal relationship of some sort between the common bile duct and the duct of Wirsung, or that when one gives glucagon there is a particular effect on the sphincter of Oddi. This must be a pharmacological action, not a physiological one.

Myren: In our series we have seen quite a lot of duodenal diverticula combined with gallstones and also with pancreatitis. I wonder, Professor McCarthy, if you have had an opportunity to test

103

manometry in such cases. As far as I know, it has been found that a higher pressure is needed to overcome the sphincter, with the result that there is often a higher frequency of bile infection with bacteria coli.

McCarthy: In my experience, with duodenal diverticuli, the passage pressure through the sphincter of Oddi is variable. I think that inflammation of the sphincter of Oddi is not uncommon with duodenal diverticuli, but it is not present with all.

Myren: I would also like to make a comment in connection with Dr Treffot's paper, and that is that I do not regard sphincter spasm as a final diagnosis in itself, but rather as a symptom of something else.

Kreel: I do not regard it as a problem in itself, and when seen it is very rarely a sign of any important underlying abnormality. My feeling is that if there is a syndrome of increased pressure at the sphincter of Oddi associated with symptoms, the diagnosis has to be made by radiomanometry, not by radiology.

Wingate: To get back to the technique described by Professor McCarthy, this certainly seems a wonderfully simple matter, but, if I have understood the data correctly, you and Dr Treffot have not come out with the same results. Dr Treffot, I believe, has found glucagon to have a relaxing effect on the sphincter of Oddi, but you have not.

McCarthy: Yes, indeed. It is a great pity that Dr Treffot is not here to discuss this point.

Paul: The thing that worries me about your technique, Professor McCarthy, simple though it may be, is that in order to use it one has to operate. Personally, whenever possible, I prefer to avoid this.

McCarthy: An operation is often unavoidable when there are stones.

Volpicelli: At the recent meeting of the American Society for Gastrointestinal Endoscopy there were three papers by American authors discussing so-called 'stenosing papillitis' (Bar-Meir, S. *et al.* (1978), *Gastrointestinal Endoscopy,* abstr., **24,** 191; Lo.Giuidice, J.A. *et al.* (1978), *Gastrointestinal Endoscopy,* abstr., **24,** 204; Zimmon, D.S. *et al.* (1978), *Gastrointestinal Endoscopy,* abstr., **24,** 214) 'Stenosing papillitis' is a diagnosis which, until now, has generally been regarded with a great deal of scepticism in the United States, but these investigators have recently developed new manometric devices which permit measurement of pressure at the sphincter of Oddi by means of endoscopic retrograde cholangiopancreatography (ERCP).

Their studies have shown that there is a group of patients with pain, with or without abnormal liver or pancreatic enzyme studies, in whom there are no demonstrable stones or other pathology, except for elevated sphincter of Oddi pressures. In an uncontrolled series they have shown that following operative sphincteroplasty or endoscopic papillotomy the elevated sphincter of Oddi pressure has returned to normal and the symptoms disappeared.

Personally I do not have much experience doing papillotomies – they are not done as often in the United States as they seem to be in some other countries, possibly because there is a lower incidence of retained common bile duct stones in the United States. As far as the diagnosis and endoscopic treatment of 'stenosing papillitis' is concerned, I have reservations about this at the moment. I hope that American endoscopists are not trying to find a use for a procedure that they have limited use for otherwise. I thought this worth reporting to you, nevertheless.

Baker: I find Professor McCarthy's data very interesting. I suggest that he and Dr Treffot are looking at different kinds of patients. I suspect that Dr Treffot's patients have papillitis, whilst Professor McCarthy's have previously undiagnosed stones. Does manometry allow one to recognize stones that would be missed radiologically? Does it add anything to the presently available radiological techniques? It would seem to me that the morbidity for the two procedures would be about the same; one has to incise the common duct for both.

McCarthy: I estimate that some 4% of common duct stones are missed by the radiologist. This is because in order to be found by the radiologist the stone must be of a certain size or must be obstructing at a very sensitive point.

Baker: Did any of your patients with normal manometry have stones?

McCarthy: Yes. Common duct stones are not incompatible with normal radiomanometry. There are free floating stones that are not associated with elevated alkaline phosphatase nor with an elevated serum bilirubin. The point of using a contrast material in manometry is to ensure that one gets a radiological image of the biliary tree, as well as determining the passage pressure through the sphincter of Oddi. In this way one has both an anatomical and a physiological measure.

8 The Role of Glucagon in the Treatment of Biliary Tract Pathology

F. Paul

Pancreatic glucagon, a polypeptide hormone of the α-cells of the islets of Langerhans, causes glycogenolysis, liberation of catecholamines, and inhibition of gastric and pancreatic secretion.[1] Relatively little interest has been shown clinically until now in the marked spasmolytic[2-11] and choleretic[2 5 12-14] effects of the hormone.

Recently, however, our group in Giessen, West Germany, using electromanometry, demonstrated a marked decrease of intraluminal bile duct pressure 20 s after the intravenous injection of 1 μg crystalline glucagon per kg bodyweight in man (Figure 8.1). Other investigators have observed a significant fall in the closing pressure of the sphincter of Oddi after glucagon

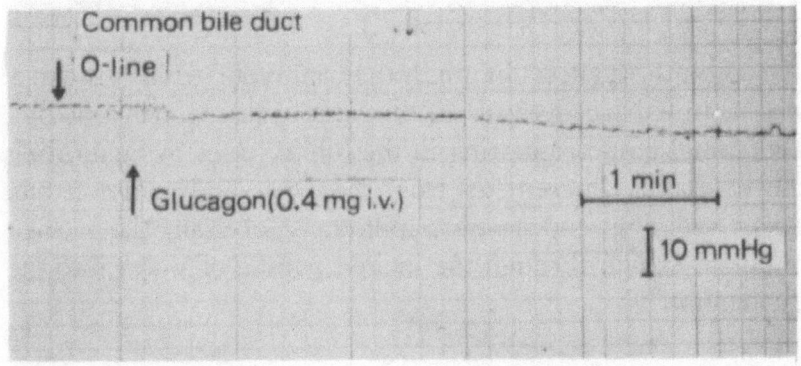

Figure 8.1 Effect of glucagon on choledochal pressure: 20 s after a single i.v. injection of 0.4 mg of glucagon a decrease of the endoluminal pressure in the common bile duct was registered reaching its maximum after 3 min 40 s (pressure registration was performed electromanometrically by means of a Statham pressure transducer (P 23 Db) and through an open-tip fluid-filled catheter which was inserted transendoscopically without premedication of the patient)

injection,[2 8] and it has also been shown that this hormone is a general inhibitor of smooth muscle tone and motility.[5 15-22] Chernish *et al.*[23] have shown that it relaxes the gallbladder and prevents its contraction being stimulated by a fatty meal, and this has also been the experience of our group (Figure 8.2).

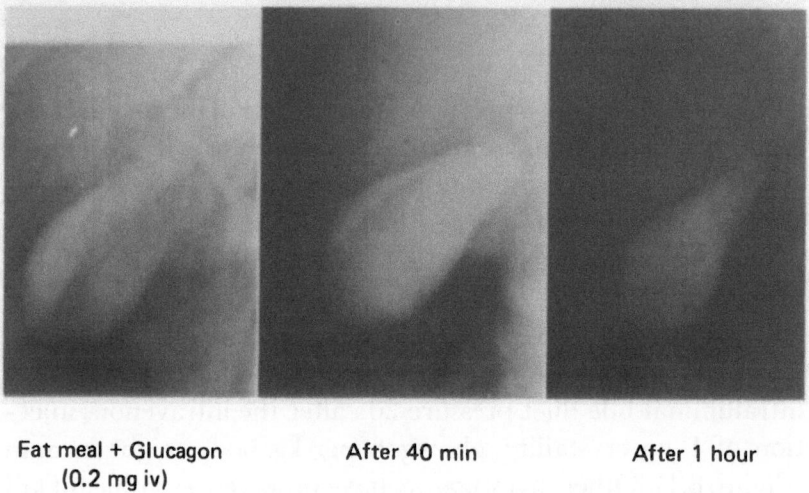

Fat meal + Glucagon   After 40 min   After 1 hour
(0.2 mg iv)

Figure 8.2 Cholecystography demonstrates that i.v. injection of glucagon inhibits the contraction of the gallbladder after a fat meal up to one hour

With these effects in mind, the trial reported in this paper was instituted in order to assess the value of glucagon in relieving abdominal pain originating in the biliary tract by facilitating the release of concrements from the cystic and common bile ducts, and, after endoscopic papillotomy, of easing the passage of ductal calculi through the incised papilla of Vater into the duodenum.

SUBJECTS AND METHODS

In this trial there were two groups of patients. One (group A) received only an intravenous bolus injection of glucagon, and the other (group B) was treated with long-term (up to 12 days) constant intravenous infusion.

Group A

The first group consisted of 31 patients (23 female and 8 male, aged 23 to 71, with a mean age of 42.6 years) suffering from acute right upper abdominal pain. Cholelithiasis was confirmed as the cause of the colic by X-ray examination and by laboratory tests. The patients in this group were given an intravenous bolus injection of 0.2 to 1 mg crystalline pancreatic glucagon. The time taken for the pain to be relieved was carefully recorded.

Group B

The second group consisted of 71 patients (60 female and 11 male, aged 18 to 92, with a mean age of 56.3 years). All these patients had concrements in the biliary tract. In 61 of these patients endoscopic papillotomy for choledocholithiasis had been performed and an additional five, each, had a stone obstruction of the cystic duct or a small concrement in the common bile duct after cholecystectomy. All 71 patients in this group received an initial intravenous bolus loading dose of 1 mg glucagon, and were then constantly infused for between 2 and 12 days with a dose of 3–5 mg glucagon per 24 hours. Subjective side effects were noted daily by the patients and by the supervising medical personnel, and blood glucose levels were measured every second day.

RESULTS

Group A

The effect of a single intravenous injection of glucagon on biliary colic pain is shown in Table 8.1. After 0.2 mg of the hormone 7 out of 10 patients became free from pain within 20 seconds to 5 minutes. Three needed additional anticholinergic-type spasmolytics for complete relief.

A dose of 0.5 mg was successful in suppressing pain in 15 out of 17 patients. In one additional patient a lasting effect was achieved upon adjunct therapy with 30 mg pentazocine. In the other, recurrent right upper abdominal colics could not be permanently suppressed by the intravenously injected

TABLE 8.1 Effect of intravenous injection of various doses of glucagon upon abdominal pain originating from biliary tree

Glucagon (mg)	Patients (n)	Painfree within 20 sec – 5 min
0.2	10	7
0.5	17	15 + 1*
1.0	4	4

*Plus pentazocine (30 mg intravenously)

glucagon, nor by the additional administration of pentazocine (30 mg) or of hyoscine butyl bromide (40 mg). When the X-ray diagnosis of cystic duct obstruction was made in this case (see Figure 8.3) intravenous infusion of 5 mg glucagon per 24 hours was initiated. During this time the patient was without pain for 2 days, but then had a recurrence of biliary colic accompanied by biochemical evidence of cholestasis with marked elevation of alkaline phosphatase and γ-glutamyl-transpeptidase levels. Upon a second course of glucagon infusion, which lasted 8 days, the patient became asymptomatic, with normalization of the enzymes and of the intravenous cholecysto-cholangiogram. It would appear that the cause of the colic in this patient was a small concrement obstructing the cystic duct, and which, during glucagon infusion, passed into the gut.

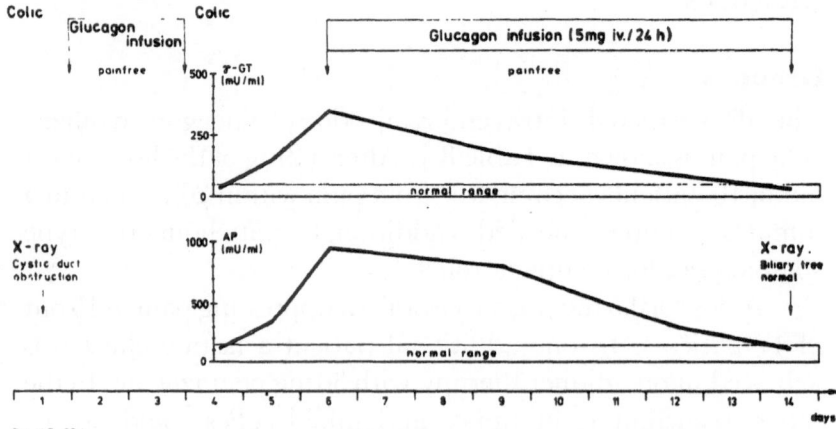

Figure 8.3 Effect of intravenous glucagon infusion in biliary colic.

A prompt relief from pain was noted in all four of the patients who received 1 mg glucagon.

Group B

The results in the 71 patients who received long-term glucagon infusion are illustrated in Figure 8.4. In 3 cases out of 5 a stone obstruction in the cystic duct was successfully resolved; similarly, in 3 of the 5 patients with choledocholithiasis and an intact papilla of Vater a small stone was released from the common bile duct making surgery unnecessary (see Figure 8.5). The other 4 patients had to be operated upon.

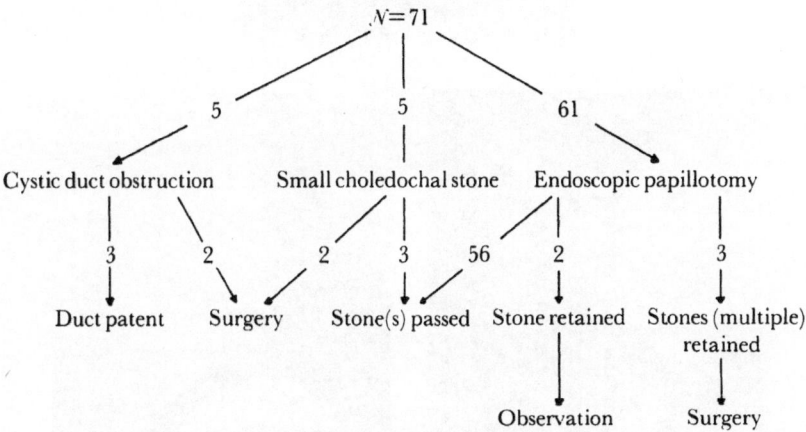

Figure 8.4 Patients treated with i.v. long-term glucagon infusion

Choledocholithiasis was successfully treated by endoscopic papillotomy followed by intravenous long-term glucagon infusion in 56 of the 61 patients treated. In 2 cases a concrement was retained, but cholestasis and cholangitis subsided promptly. These patients remain under observation. Only 3 patients had to be operated upon because endoscopic papillotomy, followed by glucagon infusion for between 7 and 12 days, was unsuccessful in clearing the common bile duct of multiple concrements. In one of these a bile duct carcinoma with a concrement incarcerated in the tumour was found during the operation.

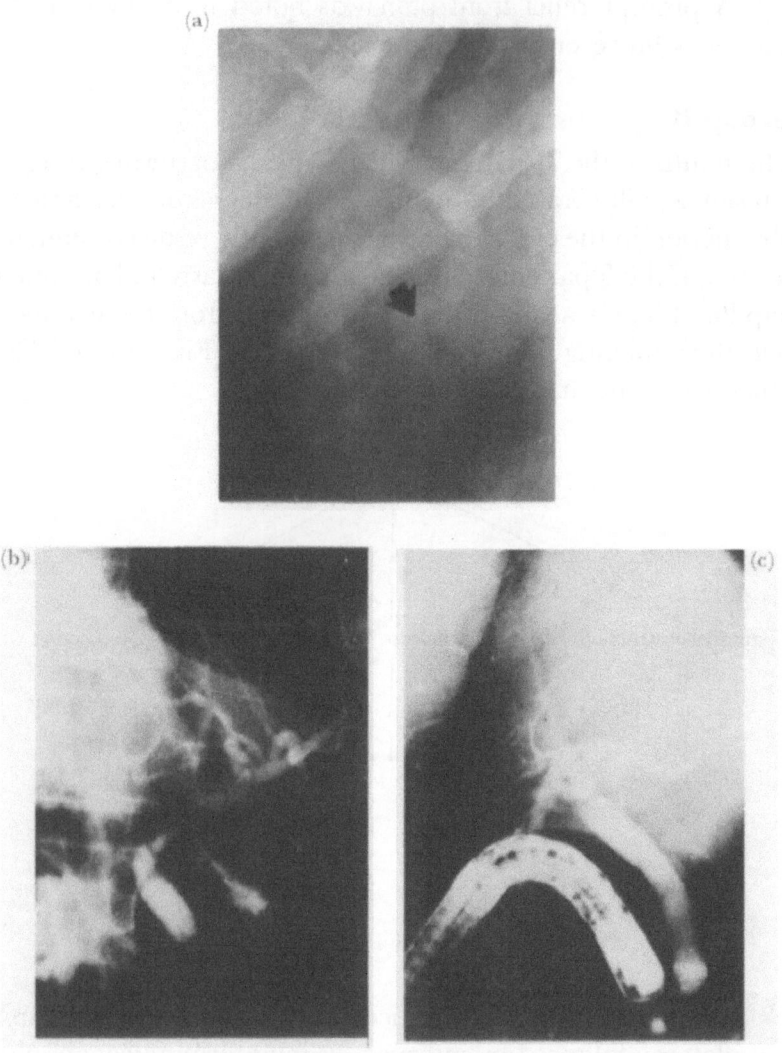

Figure 8.5 (a) Intravenous cholangiogram shows singular pre-papillary concrement (0.5 cm diam.) in the common bile duct (R. A. 67 years); (b) Same patient: concrement found in the stools after having passed the intact papilla of Vater during glucagon infusion (5 mg per 24 hours) for 4 days; (c) Same patient: endoscopic retrograde cholangiography shows the common bile duct free of concrements

SIDE EFFECTS

A single injection of 0.2–1 mg glucagon caused no side effects. In the group of patients treated with long-term infusion of the hormone, nausea and vomiting as signs of overdosage occurred in 10% of the patients ($n = 7$) but subsided when the daily dose of the hormone was reduced by one-third. An elevation of the blood glucose level by about 50% of the initial value was a regular finding.

DISCUSSION

It is well established that pancreatic glucagon has general spasmolytic and gastrointestinal motility-inhibiting properties.[4 6 7 9 10 15-24] In addition, this hormone decreases the choledochal[5 11] and sphincter of Oddi pressure,[5 8] obviously by relaxation of the smooth muscle cells scattered throughout the wall of the common bile duct and of the muscular network of the papilla of Vater, and stimulates bile flow[5 12 13] and bile salt secretion.[14] Due to these effects glucagon would theoretically seem to be of clinical therapeutic value in suppressing biliary colic pain, in resolving stone obstruction of the cystic duct and, in choledocholithiasis, in enhancing the passage of a small concrement through the intact papilla of Vater or of larger stones after endoscopic papillotomy.

It was observed that a single intravenous injection of 0.2-1 mg glucagon resulted in pain relief within 20 seconds to 5 minutes in 84% of the patients suffering from biliary colic. In this dose range glucagon elicited no side effects. It has been observed, however, that 2 mg glucagon, if not administered in divided doses or by intravenous infusion, occasionally causes nausea and vomiting.[10 20]

Constant long-term infusion of the hormone proved effective in 3 out of 5 cases of stone obstruction of the cystic duct and in a similar number of cases of choledocholithiasis when the papilla of Vater was intact. Besides favourable anatomical configuration of the papilla, the size of the concrement is obviously an important factor. In cases of choledocholithiasis with an intact papilla of Vater the stones passing spontaneously were all less than 5 mm in diameter, whilst those which had to be removed surgically were larger.

The question arises as to whether the release of the choledochal stone into the duodenum was due to the choleretic and smooth muscle relaxing effects of glucagon or was a spontaneous event. In patients with acute pancreatitis it has been found that the spontaneous passage of small choledochal concrements through the intact papilla of Vater is not at all rare. In our cases, however, the coincidence between glucagon infusion and stone release appeared to be obvious. An answer to the same question is even more difficult in those patients with choledocholithiasis in whom endoscopic papillotomy followed by glucagon infusion was successful. From theoretical considerations and the large number – compared to the literature[25] – of 92% of the patients being completely cured after these measures, long-term application of glucagon probably exerts a beneficial effect upon the course of choledocholithiasis after endoscopic papillotomy. A prospective double-blind trial would really be necessary to prove this assumption, but this is not feasible, firstly because several parameters (size, shape, and number of stones, configuration of the common bile duct, length of the incision) influence the result, and, secondly, because repeated X-ray and endoscopic examinations during the post-papillotomy phase in order to obtain information on the release of choledochal concrements are not possible. It also cannot yet be decided whether the quick regression of cholestasis and cholangitis observed in two patients in spite of a retained choledochal concrement was the result of endoscopic papillotomy alone or whether glucagon-induced choleresis, in this respect, was of therapeutic significance too.

Long-term administration of glucagon was usually well tolerated. Moderate elevation of blood sugar level was a normal laboratory finding and evidence that an effective amount of glucagon had been administered. Nausea and vomiting occurred in 10% of the patients, but subsided upon the reduction of the daily dose of glucagon by one-third. Individual sensitivity to glucagon seems to be involved since two patients became symptomatic after only a few hours infusion of the lowest initial dose of 3 mg per 24 hours. Atropine-like spasmolytics when given in effective amounts cause more side effects than glucagon. Also, they can only be administered intermittently, and various contraindications have to be considered. Since biliary concrements of clinical importance are often encountered in geriatric patients with conditions in which the use of such substances is contraindicated (e.g., prostatic hyperplasia, glaucoma, impairment of coronary and cerebral blood flow) their use is limited. Contraindications for glucagon, however, are few. Its uncontrolled long-term infusion is contraindicated in cases of phaeochromocytoma, but brittle insulin-dependent diabetes is only a relative contraindication for the administration of this hormone in biliary tract disease.

SUMMARY

The therapeutic values of the choleretic and spasmolytic properties of pancreatic glucagon in certain diseases of the biliary tract were assessed in an open clinical trial.

Biliary colic was effectively treated in 84% of the patients treated with a single intravenous injection of 0.2–1 mg of the hormone.

Experimental intravenous infusion of 3–5 mg glucagon per 24 hours for between 2 and 12 days resulted in 6 out of 10 patients in the resolution of a stone obstruction of the cystic duct or in the passing of a small concrement from the common bile duct through the intact papilla of Vater. These patients were thus spared surgical intervention.

Following endoscopic papillotomy, long-term glucagon infusion may well aid the passage of common bile duct stones into the gut. This combination of measures was successful in 92% of the patients.

Nausea and vomiting were rare side effects, and subsided upon dose reduction. Brittle diabetes is a relative contraindication and phaeochromocytoma an absolute contraindication for the long-term administration of glucagon.

Controlled studies of the clinical therapeutic relevance of the choleretic and spasmolytic effects of glucagon in biliary tract disease are now needed.

References

1 Lefèbvre, P.J. and Unger, R.H. (eds.). (1972). *Glucagon*. (Oxford: Pergamon).

2   Andersson, K. E., Andersson, R., Hedner, P. and Persson, C. G. A. (1972). Effect of cholecystokinin on the level of cyclic AMP and on mechanical activity in the isolated sphincter of Oddi. *Life Sci.,* **11**, 723.

3   Chernish, S. M., Miller, R. E., Rosenak, B. D. and Scholz, N. E. (1972). Hypotonic duodenography with the use of glucagon. *Gastroenterology,* **63**, 392.

4   Kreel, L. (1975). Pharmaco-radiology in barium examinations with special reference to glucagon. *Br. J. Radiol.,* **48**, 691.

5   Lin, T. M. and Spray, G. F. (1969). Effect of pentagastrin, cholecystokinin, caerulein and glucagon on the choledochal resistance and bile flow in the dog. *Gastroenterology,* **56**, 1178.

6   Lowman, R. M., Belleza, N. A., Goetsch, J. B., Finkelstein, H. I., Berneike, R. R. and Rosenfield, A. T. (1977). Glucagon (letter to editor). *J. Urol.,* **118**, 128.

7   Miller, R. E., Chernish, S.M., Skucas, J., Rosenak, B.D. and Rodda, B.E. (1974). Hypotonic colon examination with glucagon. *Radiology,* **113**, 555.

8   Nebel, O. T. (1964). Endoscopic manometry: a new technique for the physiologic study of the human sphincter of Oddi. *Gastroenterology,* **66**, A164/818.

9   Paul, F., Misaki, F. and Seifert, E. (1973). Crystalline pancreatic glucagon – a new spasmolytic agent: results of comparative endoscopic and electromanometric investigations in the proximal gastrointestinal tract. *Endoscopy,* **5**, 199.

10 Paul, F. and Freyschmidt, J. (1976). Anwendung von Glukagon bei endoskopischen und röntgenologischen Untersuchungen des Gastrointesti-naltrakts. *Fortschr. Röntgenstr.,* **125**, 31.

11 Paul, F. (1976). Intravenöse Langzeitinfusion von Glukagon zur Abtreibung von Gallenwegskonkrementen. *Fortschr. Endoskopie,* pp. 161–163. (Erlangen: Perimed).

12 Dyck, W. P. and Janowitz, H. D. (1971). Effect of glucagon on hepatic bile secretion in man. *Gastroenterology,* **60**, 400.

13 Jones, R. S., Geist, R. E. and Hall, A. D. (1971). The choleretic effects of glucagon and secretin in the dog. *Gastroenterology,* **60**, 64.

14 Morris, Q. T., Sardi, G. F. and Bradley, S. E. (1967). Character of glucagon-induced choleresis. *Fed. Proc.,* **26**, 774.

15 Danford, R. O. and Davidson, A. J. (1969). The use of glucagon as a vasodilator in visceral angiography. *Radiology,* **93**, 173.

16 Fasth, S. and Hultèn, L. (1971). The effect of glucagon on intestinal motility and blood flow. *Acta Physiol. Scand.,* **83**, 169.

17 Gerlock, J. A. and Hooser, C. W. (1976). Oviduct response to glucagon during hysterosalpingography. *Radiology,* **119**, 727.

18 Jaffer, S. S., Makhlouf, G. M., Schorr, B. A. and Zfass, A. M. (1974). Nature and kinetics of inhibition of lower esophageal sphincter pressure by glucagon. *Gastroenterology,* **67**, 42.

19 Kock, N. G., Darle, N. and Dotevall, G. (1967). Inhibition of intestinal

motility in man by glucagon given intraportally. *Gastroenterology,* **53,** 88.

20　Necheles, H., Sporn, J. and Walker, L. (1966). Effect of glucagon on gastro-intestinal motility. *Am. J. Gastroenterol.,* **45,** 29.

21　Paul, F. (1972). The effect of small doses of glucagon on gastric motility. *Arch. Mal. App. Digest (France),* suppl. 61, 454 (abstract).

22　Paul, F. (1974). Quantitative Untersuchungen der Wirkung von Pankreasglukagon und Sekretin auf die Magen-Darm-Motorik mittels elektromanometrischer Simultanregistrierungen beim Menschen. *Klin. Wschr.,* **52,** 983.

23　Chernish, S. M., Miller, R. E., Rosenak, B. D. and Scholz, N. E. (1972). Effect of glucagon on size of visualized human gallbladder before and after a fat meal. *Gastroenterology,* **62,** 1218.

24　Stunkard, A. J., yan Itallie, T. B. and Reiss, B. B. (1955). The mechanism of satiety: effect of glucagon on gastric hunger contractions. *Proc. Soc. Exp. Biol. Med.,* **89,** 258.

25　Koch, H., Rösch, W., Schaffner, O. and Demling, L. (1977). Endoscopic papillotomy. *Gastroenterology,* **73,** 1393.

DISCUSSION

Kreel: May I ask about urinary calculi? Have you tried this procedure for getting rid of these stones too?

Paul: Yes, we have. When we saw that biliary colic could be treated with glucagon we tried it also in patients with urinary colic. We got very satisfactory results. This has also been the experience of Lowman who recently wrote to the Journal of Urology on this subject (*J. Urol.* (1977), **118,** 128).

Myren: I think your report on the giving of glucagon when performing papillotomy or removing calculi up to 5 mm in diameter is a very interesting and useful one. What was your success rate before you started using glucagon? We had a similar series of 70–80 patients and found it necessary to re-do the papillotomy in about 10% of cases before the stones passed. Incidentally, for removing stones we use a catheter with a small balloon, not baskets; we have had no complications with this technique, but, of course, we have had bleeding in one or two cases.

Paul: I have no comparative figures as I have used glucagon from the very beginning when doing papillotomies. I think it would be very difficult to do a control study, as one cannot check the patients every day to see whether the stones are still in place or not. I have found that manipulations using wire baskets or balloons to extract the concrements are very rarely necessary, and they can be dangerous. I usually wait for the stone to pass spontaneously.

Wingate: I am interested in your dosage regime, and, while I find the results impressive, I am a little baffled as to what is actually happening. You are giving an enormous loading dose of glucagon and that, in itself, could cause the kind of effect described. The effectiveness of that glucagon will quickly fade though, because of the half-life factor. Your subsequent doses, 5 mg per 24 hours, are very low. I wonder if data from studies on choleresis are relevant in connection with your low dose infusion. What is the rationale of your dosage scheme? Do you think both doses – the bolus injection and the infusion – are effective?

Paul: Yes, I do. When we did blood sugar measurements we saw that the level always rose to about twice the initial value. This is, I think, a parameter of whether the dose is effective or not. When a patient starts to vomit, and, with a dose of 5 mg, this happens in about 10% of patients on the second day of the infusion, the dose has to be reduced. One has to test the patient's tolerance.

Wingate: Yes, but are you seeing hyperglycaemia?

Paul: Yes, there is always hyperglycaemia.

Wingate: You have not done a random double blind trial?

Paul: No, as I have already said, it would be difficult to do such a trial because one cannot endoscope or X-ray the patient every day to check whether the stone is still there or not. I cannot say that other drugs are not as useful as glucagon. What I am saying is that with glucagon we have a substance which induces choleresis and relaxes the smooth muscle of the opened papilla. It may be that the opening becomes larger under glucagon. The results obtained with glucagon are our rationale for using it.

Wingate: I wonder why you are seeing so much nausea and vomiting. What is the mechanism of this? I wonder too why diarrhoea is not included in your list of side effects, as it is in everyone else's.

Paul: I do not think the cardiologists observed diarrhoea when they gave high doses of 4 mg per hour for up to 12 days (Van der Ark, C.R. and Reynolds, G.W. (1969). *Circulation*, **40,** 206, suppl. III). For myself,

I can only say that I have done a lot of work with glucagon and have never found the hormone to cause this problem.

Baker: Your studies are very interesting, Professor Paul. Would you tell us a little more about the patients you studied? I judge that they were not acutely ill with biliary tract obstruction, so I assume that they had stones that were free in the common bile duct, or only partially obstructing bile flow. I wonder if glucagon has any physiological or pharmacological effect here at all, since it is clear that a masked post-obstructive choleresis often occurs. You can see the dilatation of the biliary tree if you look for it by radiological means, regardless of whether any choleretic agent is given. What you see may well not be an effect of glucagon.

Paul: Yes, this is probably true of patients who are jaundiced, and suffering from a complete obstruction. Most of the patients we have treated with endoscopic papillotomy, however, just had stones and colic; they were not, or only slightly, jaundiced.

Baker: So some may have had partial obstruction?

Paul: Yes.

Baker: If you did a papillotomy the patients must have had stones in the common bile duct and not in the cystic duct.

Paul: Yes, that's right. Only in a few cases were we able to remove stones from the cystic duct after cholecystectomy.

Baker: I do not know if a post-obstructive choleresis would be expected in partial common duct obstruction. I imagine so.

Paul: I do not think that obstruction of the cystic duct would lead to choleresis.

Baker: I agree, as far as the cystic duct is concerned. I was thinking of patients with common bile duct stones.

Paul: I want to stress that most of these patients were not jaundiced. Their bilirubin levels were normal. They just had stones in the common bile duct, and they suffered from biliary colic several times a week. That is why we did a papillotomy on them.

Baker: What was the follow-up? Did stones re-form in any of these patients? Did re-stenosis occur?

Paul: We started doing endoscopic papillotomies three years ago, and have since followed all patients. There have been no signs of cholangitis so far, no re-formation of stones, and no re-stenosis of the ostium. The situation is completely different when one performs an endoscopic papillotomy than when one does a choledocho-duodeno-stomy, after which we find many patients showing intermittent obstruction with cholangitis due to food particles, and so on. When we realized the lack of severe side effects of glucagon we tried to remove stones this way. We thought there might be some risk of the older patients – those in their eighties and nineties – developing cholangitis or re-stenosis, but this has not happened.

McCarthy: I am wondering if you have not discovered something important about the physiology of the gallbladder as opposed to the physiology of the sphincter of Oddi. You said, did you not, that glucagon seems to increase the size of the gallbladder. Is that right?

Paul: What we found was that 40 minutes after 0.5 mg glucagon and a fatty meal the gallbladder was not contracted; after one hour it was. I would say, therefore, that glucagon inhibits the contraction of the gallbladder after a fatty meal for something less than one hour.

McCarthy: Very good. A second question then. Have you used glucagon in an attempt to establish the differential diagnosis between acute pancreatitis and biliary colic, which is often a problem in the emergency room before the serum amylase levels are returned? Judging by your data, it would seem that a single injection of glucagon would allow the emergency room physician to make a diagnosis within one minute.

Paul: I would not go so far as to say that. We have never tried glucagon for this purpose. We have used it when we thought that a patient's pain could be due to a stone in the biliary tree, and we have then treated him with glucagon hoping that it would allow a small stone to pass into the gut. This can indeed be achieved in the occasional patient with a small ductal concrement.

9 Hepatotrophic Effects of Insulin and Glucagon and their Potential Role in the Treatment of Hepatic Failure

N. A. Volpicelli

INTRODUCTION

Disorders of the liver, particularly alcohol-related cirrhosis, are a major cause of death throughout the world and the incidence is rising.[1] Currently available therapies have done little to improve the overall survival of patients with fulminant hepatitis due to viruses, alcohol or other toxins.[2-4] In addition, merely treating the complications of chronic liver disease, such as portacaval shunt operations for bleeding oesophageal varices, does not appear to increase survival since the majority of these patients subsequently die of hepatic failure.[5 6] Unless a significant impact is made in preventing liver disease, new forms of therapy are necessary to increase survival of patients with acute and chronic liver failure.

Recent animal studies indicate that portal venous blood and its contained hormones, insulin and glucagon, are hepatotrophic.[7-39] In view of these reports, it has been suggested that insulin and glucagon may have beneficial properties in treating human hepatic failure.[40-42] The purpose of the following discussion is to review the evidence that insulin and glucagon are hepatotrophic and that the potential exists for utilizing these hormones in the treatment of human hepatic failure.

EVIDENCE SUPPORTING THE HEPATOTROPHIC QUALITIES OF INSULIN AND GLUCAGON

In 1920 Rous and Larimore[43] demonstrated that ligation of the portal venous supply to the main lobe of the rabbit liver resulted in rapid atrophy of this lobe and hypertrophy of the remaining liver tissue. In these experiments the hepatic artery and bile ducts were kept intact. They postulated that there were substances in the portal blood necessary to maintain hepatic growth. Subsequent studies confirmed the importance of portal blood since diversion of portal blood flow led to inhibition of normal hepatic regeneration following partial hepatectomy in the dog[44 45] and rat.[46] However, liver regeneration in the partially hepatectomized dog would occur if blood supply was maintained by portacaval transposition[47] or by arterialization of the hepatic end of the portal vein (by means of a jugular venous graft from the aorta) after an end-to-side portacaval shunt.[48] These studies were taken as evidence that portal venous blood was not necessary for liver regeneration and that the quantity of blood flow to the liver rather than its content was the most important factor in regeneration.

The idea that portal venous blood contained hepatotrophic factors was revived after a number of years with studies on liver transplantation. Starzl *et al.*[7] and Marchioro *et al.*[8] found that canine auxiliary homografts (liver transplantation done without removal of the host's own liver) would atrophy unless they received splanchnic blood. This atrophy occurred in the absence of splanchnic blood regardless of immunosuppressive therapy and maintenance of adequate systemic venous blood flow to the homograft. Furthermore, partial portacaval transposition (where either the right or left portal vein is anastomosed to the vena cava leaving the other attached to the main portal trunk) resulted in atrophy of that portion of the liver receiving systemic venous blood while the liver receiving portal blood hypertrophied.[9]

More evidence that portal venous blood contains hepatotrophic substances came from further studies of auxiliary liver transplants in rats,[11-14] that demonstrated the necessity of portal blood to induce significant DNA synthesis in the homograft. In addition, it was also demonstrated in rats, by means of cross-circulation experiments,[10] that partial hepatectomy in one animal would induce DNA synthesis in the liver of the non-hepatectomized partner, and this hypertrophy was further enhanced by portacaval shunt indicating that the hepatotrophic substance was in greatest concentration in the portal blood.

The majority of studies indicate that the pancreas is the major source of the hepatotrophic factors[16 18 20 37] in portal blood and that the specific factors of greatest importance are insulin and glucagon.[17 19 20-28 31 32 34-39] However, considerable controversy exists regarding these conclusions since other studies suggest that hepatotrophic factors emanate from splanchnic viscera other than the pancreas[29 30] and that there are hepatotrophic substances in the pancreas other than insulin and glucagon.[49] In this regard, it is important to note that hepatic regeneration (measured by DNA synthesis) occurs in the partially hepatectomized dog and rat even after splanchnic evisceration.[15 50] Regenerative capability is, however, considerably delayed and less pronounced in the rat following splanchnic evisceration but can be restored toward normal with glucagon and insulin.[17 22 23 25 34 35]

Controversy also exists regarding the relative importance of glucagon versus insulin. Starzl's studies in dogs[20 24 27 32 36] with alloxan-induced diabetes and total pancreatectomy indicate that insulin is the most important hepatotrophic substance in portal blood and that the role of glucagon is negligible. On the other hand, studies in partially hepatectomized eviscerated rats indicate that insulin and glucagon act synergistically to promote maximal hepatic DNA synthesis and neither hormone alone has any appreciable effect.[23 25 31 34 35] Furthermore, Price and coworkers have shown that high concentrations of insulin retard DNA synthesis in the partially hepatectomized eviscerated rat while low concentrations of insulin combined with high concentrations of glucagon permit maximal DNA synthesis.[34] This is in keeping with the observation that insulin levels in blood decline while glucagon levels rise in non-eviscerated rats with normal liver regeneration following partial hepatectomy.[28 33] Glucagon alone is generally thought to lead to catabolic events in the liver[51 52] while insulin alone appears to be anabolic.[53 54] With regard to positive hepatotrophic influences in the rat, they appear to be synergistic. The reasons for this apparent synergism are speculative.[22 23 25 28 31 34 35 37 40 55]

That the pancreatic hormones insulin and glucagon are hepatotrophins is in keeping with current thoughts that the growth of mammalian cells is under the control of polypeptide hormones.[56] The reason that initial studies were able to demonstrate hepatic growth[47 48] in the absence of a direct portal blood supply is probably the fact that liver was receiving portal hepatotrophic substances from systemic venous blood. In the cross-circulation experiment, for example, hepatotrophic factors contained in systemic blood from the partially hepatectomized animal were able to induce DNA synthesis in the non-hepatectomized partner. However, when two livers must compete for hepatotrophic factors (as in the auxiliary liver transplant studies) it appears that the concentration of portal factors in systemic blood is too low to maintain growth. From the foregoing, Rous and Larimore's postulate regarding hepatotrophic substances in portal blood appears to be correct and the quantity of blood flow to the liver is less important than its content. Differences of opinion regarding the specific source and factors that are hepatotrophic are most likely accounted for by the different animal species and experimental models used in the studies. Furthermore, there appear to be other hormonal substances that have hepatotrophic properties.[57]

None of the foregoing discussion should detract from the apparent importance of insulin and glucagon. Several recent studies, utilizing models of liver failure with human counterparts, have provided evidence that insulin and glucagon are potential therapeutic agents in these disorders. Farivar *et al.*[37] reported statistically significant increased survival of mice infected with murine hepatitis when given infusions of insulin and glucagon. This increase in survival occurred even if hormone infusion was delayed for 24 hours. Wands *et al.*[58] found a protective effect of glucagon and insulin on D-galactosamine liver injury in mice. Tolman and Gray[59] also found a protective effect of insulin and glucagon on salicylate-induced hepatic injury. Finally, Lindberg *et al.*[60] found that glucagon-treated rats were more efficient in reducing blood lactate levels following haemorrhagic shock. They felt this was due to improved metabolic function at the cellular level rather than changes in blood flow to the liver previously shown to occur following glucagon administration.[61]

POTENTIAL ROLE OF INSULIN AND GLUCAGON IN HUMAN HEPATIC FAILURE

Observations in humans that tend to support the above animal studies include the following:

1. Diabetics have a high incidence of cirrhosis.[62]
2. Portacaval shunts in patients with established liver disease frequently lead to an accelerated and fatal worsening of liver function.[56]
3. Portal vein obstruction impairs function in the normal liver, and this impairment increases with the duration of obstruction.[63]

In the consideration of possible human studies several potential deleterious effects of insulin and glucagon must be considered. With respect to insulin, hypoglycaemia in the patient with hepatic failure and decreased glycogen stores is a major concern. High levels of circulating glucagon may produce a 'glucagonoma' syndrome[64][65] characterized by dermatitis, weight loss, diabetes and in some cases diarrhoea. Finally, it has been suggested[66-68] that the modest hyperinsulinaemia and hyperglucagonaemia known to occur in patients with cirrhosis[69][70] leads to a decreased molar ratio of insulin to glucagon. Changes in this molar ratio are related to increases in aromatic amino acids and a decline in branched-chain amino acids in the plasma. This is thought to be a major factor in the pathogenesis of hepatic coma. Thus, any human studies must be well controlled and particular attention must be paid to the possible deleterious effects of insulin and glucagon.

Studies to date indicate that insulin and glucagon hepatotrophic effects occur during liver regeneration following hepatectomy or toxic damage. It is expected, therefore, that any benefit observed in humans would be found in disorders characterized by active inflammation and necrosis such as fulminant toxic (e.g. alcohol) or viral hepatitis. In view of this evidence and the lack of current therapy for these disorders, human studies are indicated.

CONCLUSIONS

1. It would appear from animal studies that the content of blood reaching the liver is more important than the quantity of blood in regard to hepatic regeneration and growth.

2. Hepatotrophic factors in portal venous blood appear to arise from the pancreas. Glucagon and insulin appear to be the most important factors.

3. Hepatic regeneration can occur in the absence of glucagon and insulin but is delayed and less pronounced as measured by DNA synthesis.

4. The relative importance of insulin versus glucagon with regard to their trophic influences on the liver is still controversial. Most studies to date indicate that they act synergistically.

5. The beneficial effects that glucagon and insulin may have for human hepatic failure should be studied.

References

1 Massé, L., Juillan, J. M. and Chisloup, A. (1976). Trends in mortality from cirrhosis of the liver. *World Health Statistics Report*, **29,** 40.

2 Gregory, P. B., Knauer, C. M., Kempson, R. L. *et al.* (1976). Steroid therapy in severe viral hepatitis. Double-blind randomized trial of methyl-prednisolone versus placebo. *N. Engl. J. Med.*, **294,** 681.

3 Conn, H. O. (1978). Steroid treatment of alcoholic hepatitis. *Gastroenterology,* **74,** 319.

4 Sherlock, S. (1975). Acute (fulminant) hepatic failure. In S. Sherlock, (ed.). *Diseases of the Liver and Biliary System,* 5th ed., pp. 107–121. (Oxford: Blackwell Scientific Publications).

5 Conn, H. O., Lindenmuth, W. W., May, C. J. *et al.* (1972). Prophylactic portacaval anastomosis. *Medicine,* **51,** 27.

6 Resnick, R. H., Iber, F. L., Ishihara, A. M. *et al.* (1974). Controlled study of the therapeutic portacaval shunt. *Gastroenterology,* **67,** 843.

7 Starzl, T. E., Marchioro, T. L., Rowlands, D. T. Jr. *et al.* (1964). Immunosuppression after experimental and clinical homotransplantation of the liver. *Ann. Surg.,* **160,** 411.

8 Marchioro, T. L., Porter, K. A., Dickinson, T. C. *et al.* (1965). Physiologic requirements for auxiliary liver homotransplanation. *Surg. Gynec. Obstet.,* **121,** 17.

9 Marchioro, T. L., Porter, K. A., Brown, B. I. *et al.* (1967). Effect of partial portacaval transposition on the canine liver. *Surgery,* **61,** 723.

10 Fisher, B., Szuch, P., Levine, M. *et al.* (1971). Portal blood factor as the humoral agent in liver regeneration. *Science,* **171,** 575.

11 Fisher, B., Szuch, P. and Fisher, E. R. (1971). Evaluation of a humoral factor in liver regeneration utilizing liver transplants. *Cancer Res.,* **31,** 322.

12 Lee, S., Chandler, J. G., Williams, R. *et al.* (1971). Trophic factor in portal blood required for liver regeneration. *Gastroenterology,* **60,** 688.

13 Chandler, J. G., Lee, S., Krubel, R. *et al.* (1971). Inter-liver competition and portal blood in regeneration of auxiliary liver transplants. *Surg. Forum,* **22,** 341.

14 Orloff, M. J., Lee, S., Chandler, J. G. *et al.* (1972). Humoral regulation of liver regeneration by a hepatotrophic portal blood factor. *Gastroenterology,* **62,** 791.

15 Max, M. H., Price, J. B., Takeshige, K. *et al.* (1972). Role of factors of portal origin in modifying hepatic regeneration. *J. Surg. Res.,* **12,** 120.

16 Lee, S., Duguay, L. R. and Orloff, M. J. (1972). Pancreas extract and liver regeneration. *Surg. Forum,* **27,** 358.

17 Price, J. B. Jr., Takeshige, K., Max, M. H. *et al.* (1972). Glucagon as the portal factor modifying hepatic regeneration. *Surgery,* **72,** 74.

18 Sgro, J. C., Charters, A. C., Chandler, J. G. *et al.* (1973). Site of origin of the hepatotrophic portal blood factor involved in liver regeneration. *Surg. Forum,* **24,** 377.

19 Whittemore, A. D., Kasuya, M., Fodor, P. B. *et al.* (1973). Hepatic regeneration in the rat without portal organs. *Surg. Forum,* **24,** 384.

20 Starzl, T. E., Francavilla, A., Halgrimson, C. G. *et al.* (1973). Origin, hormonal nature, and action of hepatotrophic substances in portal venous blood. *Surg. Gynecol. Obstet.,* **137,** 179.

21 Ozawa, K., Yamaoka, Y., Nanbu, H. *et al.* (1974). Insulin as the primary factor governing changes in mitochondrial metabolism leading to liver regeneration and atrophy. *Am. J. Surg.,* **127,** 669.

22 Whittemore, A. D., Kasuya, M., Voorhees, A. B. Jr. *et al.* (1975). Hepatic regeneration in the absence of portal viscera. *Surgery,* **77,** 419.

23 Bucher, N. L. R. and Swaffield, M. N. (1975). Regulation of hepatic regeneration in rats by synergistic action of insulin and glucagon. *Proc. Natl. Acad. Sci. USA,* **72,** 1157.

24 Starzl, T. E., Porter, K. A., Kashiwagi, N. *et al.* (1975). Effect of diabetes mellitus on portal blood hepatotrophic factors in dogs. *Surg. Gynecol. Obstet.,* **140,** 549.

25 Bucher, N. L. R. and Swaffield, M. N. (1975). Synergistic action of glucagon and insulin in regulation of hepatic regeneration. *Adv. Enzyme Regul.,* **13,** 281.

26 Starzl, T. E., Porter, K. A., Kashiwagi, N. *et al.* (1975). Portal hepatotrophic factors, diabetes mellitus and acute atrophy, hypertrophy and regeneration. *Surg. Gynecol. Obstet.,* **141,** 843.

27 Starzl, T. E., Porter, K. A., and Putnam, C. W. (1975). Intraportal insulin protects from the liver injury of portacaval shunt in dogs. *Lancet,* **ii,** 1241.

28 Bucher, N. L. R. (1976). Insulin, glucagon, and the liver. *Adv. Enzyme Regul.*, **15,** 221.

29 Chandler, J. G. (1976). Hepatotrophic activity in nonpancreatic, non-duodenal portal blood. *Surg. Forum*, **27,** 360.

30 Sakai, A., Pfeffermann, R., Taha, M. *et al.* (1976). Origin of regeneration factor. *Surg. Forum*, **27,** 45.

31 Whittemore, A. D., Voorhees, A. B. Jr. and Price, J. B. Jr. (1976). Hepatic blood flow and pancreatic hormones as modifiers of hepatic regeneration. *Surg. Forum*, **27,** 363.

32 Starzl, T. E., Watanabe, K., Porter, K. A. *et al.* (1976). Effects of insulin, glucagon, and insulin/glucagon infusions on liver morphology and cell division after complete portacaval shunt in dogs. *Lancet*, **i,** 821.

33 Rosenkranz, E., Duguay, L. R. and Orloff, M. J. (1976). Effect of liver regeneration on pancreatic hormone levels in blood. *Gastroenterology*, **70,** 991.

34 Price, J. B. (1976). Insulin and glucagon as modifiers of DNA synthesis in the regenerating rat liver. *Metabolism*, **25,** (suppl. 1), 1427.

35 Bucher, N. L. R. and Weir, G. C. (1976). Insulin, glucagon, liver regeneration, and DNA synthesis. *Metabolism*, **25,** (suppl. 1), 1423.

36 Starzl, T. E., Porter, K. A. and Putnam, C. W. (1976). Insulin, glucagon and the control of hepatic structure, function, and capacity for regeneration. *Metabolism*, **25,** (suppl. 1), 1429.

37 Farivar, M., Wands, J. R., Isselbacher, K. J. *et al.* (1976). Effect of insulin and glucagon on fulminant murine hepatitis. *N. Engl. J. Med.*, **295,** 1517.

38 Duguay, L. R., Skivolocki, W. P., Lee, S. *et al.* (1977). Regulation of liver regeneration by pancreatic hormones. *Gastroenterology*, **72,** 1053.

39 Yamada, T., Yamamoto, M., Ozawa, K. *et al.* (1977). Insulin requirements for hepatic regeneration following hepatectomy. *Ann. Surg.*, **185,** 35.

40 Popper, H. (1974). Implications of portal hepatotrophic factors in hepatology. *Gastroenterology*, **66,** 1227.

41 Editorial (1975). Insulin and the liver. *Lancet*, **ii,** 1245.

42 Sherlock, S. (1976). Portal venous 'goodies' and fulminant viral hepatitis. *N. Engl. J. Med.*, **295,** 1535.

43 Rous, P. and Larimore, L. D. (1920). Relation of the portal blood to liver maintenance. A demonstration of liver atrophy conditional on compensation. *J. Exp. Med.*, **31,** 609.

44 Mann, F. C., Fishback, F. C., Gay, J. G. *et al.* (1931). Experimental pathology of the liver. Studies III, IV, and V. *Arch. Pathol.*, **12,** 787.

45 Mann, F. C. (1940). The portal circulation and restoration of the liver after partial removal. *Surgery*, **8,** 225.

46 Stephenson, G. W. (1932). Experimental pathology of the liver. IX. Restoration of the liver after partial hepatectomy and partial ligation of the portal vein. *Arch. Pathol.*, **14,** 484.

47 Child, C. G. III, Barr, D., Holswade, G. R. *et al.* (1953). Liver regeneration following portacaval transposition in dogs. *Ann. Surg.*, **138,** 600.

48 Fisher, B., Russ, C., Updegraff, H. *et al.* (1954). Effect of increased hepatic blood flow upon liver regeneration. *Arch. Surg.,* **69,** 263.

49 Skivolocki, W. P. and Orloff, M. J. (1978). Stimulation of liver regeneration by pancreatic hepatotrophic factors other than insulin and glucagon. *Gastroenterology,* **74,** 1097.

50 Bucher, N. L. R. and Swaffield, M. N. (1973). Regeneration of liver in rats in the absence of portal splanchnic organs and a portal blood supply. *Cancer Res.,* **33,** 3189.

51 Amherdt, M., Harris, V., Renold, A. E. *et al.* (1974). Hepatic autophagy in uncontrolled experimental diabetes and its relationships to insulin and glucagon. *J. Clin. Invest.,* **54,** 188.

52 Deter, R. L. (1975). Analog modeling of glucagon-induced autophagy in rat liver. I – Conceptual and mathematical model of telolysosome–auto-phagosome–autolysosome interaction. *Exp. Cell Res.,* **94,** 122.

53 Younger, L. R., King, J. and Steiner, D. F. (1966). Hepatic proliferative response to insulin in severe alloxan diabetes. *Cancer Res.,* **26,** 1408.

54 Reaven, E. P., Peterson, D. T. and Reaven, G. M. (1973). Effect of experimental diabetes mellitus and insulin replacement on hepatic ul-trastructure and protein synthesis. *J. Clin. Invest.,* **52,** 248.

55 Leffert, H. L., Koch, K. S. and Rubalcava, B. (1976). Present paradoxes in the environmental control of hepatic proliferation. *Cancer Res.,* **36,** 4250.

56 Holley, R. W. (1975). Control of growth of mammalian cells in cell culture. *Nature,* **258,** 487.

57 Richman, R. A., Claus, T. H., Pilkis, S. J. *et al.* (1976). Hormonal stimula-tion of DNA synthesis in primary cultures of adult rat hepatocytes. *Proc. Natl. Acad. Sci. USA,* **73,** 3589.

58 Wands, J. R., Storer, R., Patel, U. *et al.* (1977). Pancreatic hormonal influence on D-galactosamine induced acute liver cell injury. *Gastro-enterology,* **73,** 1253.

59 Tolman, K. G. and Gray, P. (1978). Protective effect of insulin and glucagon in salicylate hepatotoxicity. *Clin. Res.,* **26,** 114A.

60 Lindberg, B., Haljamäe, H., Jonsson, O. *et al.* (1978). Effect of glucagon and blood transfusion on liver metabolism in hemorrhagic shock. *Ann. Surg.,* **187,** 103.

61 Krarup, N. and Larsen, J. A. (1974). The effect of glucagon on hepatosplanchnic hemodynamics, functional capacity, and metabolism of the liver in cats. *Acta Physiol. Scand.,* **91,** 42.

62 Creutzfeldt, W., Frerichs, H. and Sickinger, K. (1970). Liver diseases and diabetes mellitus. In H. Popper and F. Shaffner, (eds.). *Progress in Liver Diseases,* pp. 371–407. (New York: Grune and Stratton).

63 Thompson, E. N., Williams, R. and Sherlock, S. (1964): Liver function in extrahepatic portal hypertension. *Lancet,* **ii,** 1352.

64 Mallinson, C. N., Bloom, S. R., Warin, A. P. *et al.* (1974). A glucagonoma syndrome. *Lancet,* **ii,** 1.

65 Boden, G., Owen, O. E., Rezvani, I. *et al.* (1977). An islet cell carcinoma

containing glucagon and insulin. Chronic glucagon excess and glucose homeostasis. *Diabetes,* **26,** 128.

66 Munro, H. N., Fernstrom, J. D. and Wurtman, R. J. (1976). Insulin, plasma aminoacid imbalance, and hepatic coma. *Lancet,* **i,** 722.

67 Soeters, P. B. and Fischer, J. E. (1976). Insulin, glucagon, amino acid imbalance, and hepatic encephalopathy. *Lancet,* **ii,** 880.

68 Soeters, P. B., Weir, G., Ebeid, A. M. *et al.* (1977). Insulin, glucagon, portal systemic shunting, and hepatic failure in the dog. *J. Surg. Res.,* **23,** 183.

69 Sherwin, R., Joshi, P., Hendler, R. *et al.* (1974). Hyperglucagonaemia in Laennec's cirrhosis. The role of portal-systemic shunting. *N. Engl. J. Med.,* **290,** 239.

70 Shurberg, J. L., Resnick, R. H., Koff, R. S. *et al.* (1977). Serum lipids, insulin, and glucagon after portacaval shunt in cirrhosis. *Gastroenterology,* **72,** 301.

DISCUSSION

Volpicelli: Before we begin this discussion I should like to introduce Dr Baker and Dr Jaspan from the Department of Medicine at the University of Chicago. Dr Baker and Dr Jaspan have clinical experience with glucagon and insulin and are using these substances in the treatment of a rather fulminating type of hepatic failure, namely alcoholic hepatitis. I have asked them to tell us something about their work, particularly about the study in which they are engaged at the present time. I personally have not yet used these drugs in the treatment of hepatitis, but am looking forward to doing so in the near future.

Myren: You have presented a very interesting review of the various hepatotrophic agents. Do you know if any effect has been seen on the pancreas either in animals or in man? I seem to remember that some groups have felt that the cholecystokinin effect might increase the volume and weight of the pancreas, and that this might affect the pancreatic secretion. Do you know if, in the studies you reviewed, any effects have been seen on the pancreas or on any other organs of the abdomen, on the small intestine perhaps, or was it only the liver that was hypertrophied?

Volpicelli: In the studies I reviewed it was the liver which was concentrated upon, and it was not mentioned if changes in other organs were observed.

Chairman: At this stage perhaps Dr Baker or Dr Jaspan would be so kind as to tell us about the study they are working on in Chicago.

Baker: The study being done utilizing insulin and glucagon infusions in alcoholic hepatitis patients at the University of Chicago is multidisciplinary, involving the Liver Study Unit and Endocrinology and General Medicine sections of the Department of Medicine. In addition, our Biomedical Computation Facility has been involved in design of the randomization scheme and in data analysis. After giving informed written consent, patients are randomized by sealed envelope to receive insulin and glucagon or dextrose in water. Infusions contain either 24 units of insulin and 2400 μg of glucagon in 200 ml of dextrose with albumin to prevent absorption of the hormones to infusion apparatus or 200 ml of dextrose in water with albumin added, so that the solutions cannot be distinguished by sight. Patients are infused with the solutions during the daytime for 12 hours over 3 weeks for easy supervision of therapy. Two patients early in our study became hypoglycaemic, so we now monitor blood sugar levels meticulously in all patients. Subsequently, we have had no further problems with blood sugar control. We have not seen any complications which we think are directly attributable to glucagon infusion, although a few patients have developed a paralytic ileus. However, these individuals were extremely ill and the ileus subsided with continued infusion. Some patients developed rashes, but these were not typical of the dermatitis described in the glucagonoma syndrome.

We have treated 31 patients to date, and the mean serum bilirubin level in our control and insulin and glucagon treated groups is similar, indicating adequate randomization of patients. In addition, the death rate in this initial group of patients is approximately 25%, indicating that we are dealing with a very ill patient population, similar to that described in other studies of severe alcoholic liver disease treated in university medical centres (Hardison, W..G. and Lee, F.I. (1966). *N. Engl. J. Med.*, **275**, 61). The elevated insulin and glucagon levels measured in treated patients indicate that the infusion technique is effective. All patients are evaluated systematically for clinical features and liver function tests during the three weeks of infusion. Our statistician knows which patients receive the active infusion, but all we clinicians can say at the moment is that some patients have improved and others have deteriorated. We are most interested in documenting significantly less mortality in treated patients, however.

The study of liver regeneration is an important but extremely complex and difficult area, and there are certainly other hepatotrophic factors besides glucagon and insulin. Recent evidence indicates that epidermal growth stimulating factor might be the actual initiating hormone in this process (Bucher, N.L. *et al.* (1977). In *Hepatotrophic Factors,* pp. 95–110, New York: Elsevier-Excerpta Medica). Other investigators have suggested that certain mixtures of amino acids can be substituted for glucagon in producing liver regeneration, providing further evidence that the process is quite complex. However, I was not very impressed with the report by Skivoloki and Orloff given at Digestive Diseases Week (May 1974) in Las Vegas. These workers injected a crude extract of pancreas into animals, so that the regeneration may simply have been related to necrosis caused by trypsin administration resulting in a burst of hepatic regeneration. Yet, further investigation of all the factors which might contribute to liver regeneration is worthwhile, because no single treatment modality now affords the clinician control of this important process.

McCarthy: Is there any suggestion that the route of administration makes any difference? Is the systemic intravenous administration equal to intraportal administration?

Baker: Dr Jaspan may be able to comment on this better than I can. Certainly the levels of insulin and glucagon which can be measured in the portal blood are very high. In the periphery there is a very significant fall in both hormones across the liver, because this organ extracts these substances. Ideally, one would like to give the hormones into the portal vein, but this is impractical.

Volpicelli: We have considered doing this in the study we are planning. The doses of glucagon and insulin that we shall give are much the same as those being given in the Chicago study, so we are anticipating that the concentrations in the portal vein will be much higher than are normally seen. It must also be remembered that many patients with portal venous hypertension have predominantly hepatopedal flow of blood, and this may adversely affect the amount of hepatotrophic substances reaching the liver if infused by means of the portal system. For these reasons we are proposing to give the drugs systemically in our study.

Jaspan: The point Professor McCarthy made about the site is a very good one, and it is clear that giving glucagon or insulin into the portal vein would be better. This highlights a very important aspect: that of diet and good nutrition. The eating of a normal meal stimulates the production of glucagon and of insulin, and even though the doses we are giving in the Chicago study are high enough to get to the portal vein in high concentrations, they may not be great enough if the effect we are after is a pharmacological one rather than a physiological one. However, even granting this, given the knowledge we have at the present time, it is not feasible to give the dose intraportally. We must, therefore, administer the hormones peripherally, but this must be backed up with good nutrition, and if the patient cannot eat it is very important that he be given adequate intravenous nutrition. Good oral nutrition is preferable in this regard since this is the best way of attaining reasonably high intraportal levels of insulin and glucagon as well as stimulating other as yet unrecognized substances which may be hepatotrophic too. This really raises the whole question of the role of nutrition in liver disease, an area about which not much is known. The possibility remains that nutrition may be beneficial in this regard, due, at least in part, to stimulation of hepatotrophic peptides.

To return to a point raised by Dr Volpicelli in his paper, one would like to know more about the signal which must be passed from the diseased or necrotic liver to the pancreas in order to cause the production of the hepatotrophic substances to be increased. One would like to know what this signal is, and how the message is transmitted. This is something that really should be looked into.

Another interesting point was raised by Dr Volpicelli when he asked how one could equate the apparently opposite actions of glucagon and insulin with a synergistic role. One must postulate that this effect is not the result of the familiar metabolic actions of the hormones. One is not dealing here with anabolism nor with catabolism of hepatic metabolites. Possibly it is a primary action on nucleoprotein synthesis, one which is completely different from present known actions. This too is something about which more needs to be known.

My final comment is about the doses. Mention has been made of 'pharmacological' and of 'physiological' doses. I must say that, in this instance, with the knowledge available, I find it difficult to know where one ends and the other begins. The doses being given in the Chicago study result in blood levels of glucagon that are usually 10–20 times normal, which should bring them into the 'pharmacological' category. The doses are, however, actually lower than those which are being used in the radiological studies we have been hearing about, and are at a level which, judging by other opinions expressed today, should certainly have resulted in effects such as choleresis, and so on, but this has not been the case. However, the insulin doses used have been relatively modest in comparison with glucagon-producing peripheral insulin levels that are in general only slightly above those that occur following a standard meal.

General Discussion

Chairman: Professor A. Oriol Bosch

Chairman: The papers presented at this workshop have dealt with the pharmacology of glucagon, its value as an aid to diagnosis in conjunction with endoscopy and radiology, and its possible uses as a therapeutic agent. In this final discussion session you are perfectly free to raise any points you wish, but there are two aspects that I should particularly like to see covered. Firstly, I think we should sum up the advantages and disadvantages of glucagon from each of our viewpoints, and, secondly, again taking advantage of the fact that we are all from different disciplines, I should like to hear what work you yourselves would like to do in this field, and also, what you would like to see each other doing: what does the surgeon think the radiologist should be doing, what does the radiologist think the endoscopist should be doing, and so on. Time and money are of little importance here; this is an exercise for our intellectual powers and for our imaginations.

Kreel: My first challenge would be to Dr Wingate and his team in London. I should like to see the electrical studies he has done in the gastrointestinal tract repeated in the genito-urinary tract. The response to pain in the genito-urinary system is similar to that in the biliary tract, and many drugs that act in the gut act in a similar way in the genito-urinary tract. It is a large field for diagnosis and for treatment, and we really know very little about the kind of electrical activity being elucidated there.

Wingate: A few people, including some at the London Hospital, are already looking at this. I think it is really a question of whether one is talking about the physiology or the pharmacology of glucagon. We have discussed this before. Is the gut the true target organ of pancreatic glucagon, or are we just looking at pharmacological effects? The same question must apply to the urinary system. I suspect that some of the effects of glucagon on the genito-urinary system are pharmacological ones, but this, of course, is no reason not to study them.

135

I should like to throw a challenge back to Dr Kreel. It seems to me that for some time now radiologists have been talking in a private language when they have spoken of 'motility' in the gut. I would like to see radiological studies becoming more 'physiological'. The radiologists, and we, should, for example, be looking at radio-opaque substances which act as different stimuli to the gut. We should be looking at nutrient radio-opaque meals. I am worried about the reliance placed at present on barium, and would like to see the radiologists moving away from this.

Kreel: In the last ten years there has indeed been a move away from physiology in radiology, and we have tended to concentrate more on detailed anatomical interpretations. There seemed to be very little correlation between transit times, the effect of different nutrients, and the possibilities of diagnosis in physiological terms, so we have tended not to continue with that work.

Chairman: Moving back to glucagon, could we perhaps summarize the situation in each of our fields?

Myren: Glucagon certainly has great value where endoscopy is concerned. It is particularly useful when quietness and decreased secretions are needed in order that small changes may be observed – for biopsy and snare resection, for instance, for polypectomies and therapeutic procedures. We know a great deal about it already, but more control studies are needed in order that we may know its true value in all respects. It certainly has advantages over atropine and anticholinergics, and is particularly valuable when one does not wish to use sedatives or anticholinergics.

Kreel: It is certainly the most harmless of all the muscle relaxants. It is a pity that it has to be given by injection. Whilst this is not a problem in most patients, by and large an oral preparation is preferred, particularly for diagnostic purposes. This is why I am interested in the possibility of arginine stimulating glucagon. Perhaps it will prove possible for a pathway such as this to be used to produce the same effects. I should like to raise another point: only the minimum effective dose of glucagon should be used, both as a cost-effective measure, and from the point of view of a more sensible utilization of the drug.

Jaspan: I agree with your comments. Glucagon is available at present in three dosage forms: 1, 2, and 10 mg. Looking at the presently used doses, especially those used in connection with endoscopy and radiology, it would seem desirable to have it packed in strengths of 0.2 and 0.4 mg as well. Your point about arginine is an interesting one, but I am afraid it would not work. This is because, although glucagon can indeed be stimulated by oral protein, arginine is extremely unpalatable and an oral dose is really not at all feasible. One could, of course, administer arginine intravenously, but then one might as well use glucagon.

Myren: What is the price of a single dose of glucagon?

Paul: In Germany the cost of a single dose of 0.5 mg glucagon is about the same as that of one ampoule of hyoscine butyl bromide.

Chairman: Moving on again, I should like Professor McCarthy to summarize the advantages and disadvantages of glucagon as far as the biliary tract is concerned.

McCarthy: It seems to me that we have not yet answered one very basic question, and that is whether the sphincter of Oddi is relaxed to a significant degree by the infusion of glucagon. I remain unconvinced that it is, and I rather feel that, physiologically, it should not be. Be that as it may, the evidence of relaxation of the sphincter of Oddi seems to me to be equivocal at best. Judging from what Professor Paul has said, I believe that glucagon may result in a relaxation of the cholecystokinin-induced spasm or contraction of the gallbladder. It might result in the opening of the valves of Heister and this may be the mechanism for the relief of colic. It is potentially exciting to think that glucagon is a choleretic agent. The idea that small concretions could be washed downstream in the choleretic flow and so encouraged to pass is an attractive hypothesis. I do not believe that anyone has said that glucagon in itself is able to treat cholecystolithiasis.

Chairman: From what we have heard, it would appear that the only contraindications are phaeochromocytoma, insulinoma, and some diabetes. Do the endocrinologists have any comments to make on the disadvantages of glucagon?

Gomez-Pan: I agree that phaeochromocytoma and insulinoma are contraindications, but I do not feel that diabetes should necessarily be regarded as one, since the glucagon can be compensated for by an increase in the insulin regime.

I have been thinking about the chemical structure of glucagon, and wonder if it might not be possible by changing this very slightly to produce an analogue which would retain the paracarbohydrate extra metabolic effect and be an active relaxant, but be easier to administer, perhaps intranasally or orally. This is, perhaps, something that the basic chemists should look into.

Jaspan: That is a very good suggestion, and, from what I have read recently, not at all beyond the bounds of possibility. Moody is one of the leading investigators in this field, and he has recently published on this subject (Moody, A.J. (1977) in *Glucagon: Its Role in Physiology and Clinical Medicine,* Foa, Bajaj, and Foa (eds.), p. 129, New York: Springer-Verlag, see also Assan, R. and Slusher, N. (1972). *Diabetes,* **21,** 843, and Sundby, F. *et al.* (1976). *Horm. Metab. Res.,* **8,** 366). In the course of his work on enteroglucagon, which is not really related to glucagon, Dr Moody has identified a molecule that is at present being called a 'pro-glucagon'. This pro-glucagon does not act exactly as glucagon does, but it seems that it, or something similar, is present both in enteroglucagon and in glucagon. It may well be that the myorelaxant activity of glucagon is, in fact, housed in just the pro-glucagon segment and not in the glucagon as a whole. I certainly agree that this is an area which should be further researched.

Wingate: This raises the whole issue of glucagon in the digestive tract. We have to know what enteroglucagon is, what releases it, what it does, and so on. There is a lot of glucagon in the gastrointestinal tract, but we do not really know why it is there, exactly what it does, nor what happens to it. If we could find some stimulus for its release we could, perhaps, put it in the portal system ourselves. Much work remains to be done on these peptides and on what they are doing in the digestive tract. I do not feel, however, that these are insoluble problems.

Gomez-Pan: It seems to me that one of the main problems at the present time is that we are not differentiating sufficiently well between the various peptides found in the gut. I have no doubt that we shall read in the papers tomorrow or next month that some new hormones have been isolated, but to really identify these hormones properly and to completely understand their actions and interactions is a very complicated matter. The most important endocrine organs are so diffusely distributed throughout the body that it is difficult to ascribe a physiological, or even pharmacological, role to each of the hormones or chemical messengers circulating. It *can* be done, however, and one of the ways of doing this, once one knows the structure of the substances concerned, is by chemical dissection using antibodies. In this way one is able to determine what the individual substances are, where they are having an effect, and what the effects are. If, for instance, one was to passively immunize animals with enteroglucagon antibody, thereby depleting the system of enteroglucagon, by noting the missing actions one would discover the effects of this particular hormone. Having identified each substance and its actions in this way, one can undertake combination studies. This is necessary as hormones always work in association with one another – sometimes positively and sometimes in a counter-regulatory fashion. In short, in order to understand the interactions of hormones, one has first to know what the substances are, then to deplete the system of each of them singly, and finally to test them in different combinations. This, to my mind, is a good physiological approach to the problem.

Myren: Four or five new peptides are to be reported at the Second International Symposium on Gastrointestinal Hormones, which is to be held shortly in Norway (since published; see Myren, J. (1978). symp. procs., *Scand. J. Gastroent.*, suppl. 49), and Professor Rehfeld from Aarhus in Denmark has recently reported that he has divided the gastrin and cholecystokinin pancreozymin molecules into separate parts and produced an antibody for each.

I should like to come back to the matter of complications or side effects of glucagon, and ask about the possible effects of long-term treatment, for, as Professor Paul has told us, it is sometimes necessary, in some cases of stones for instance, to administer glucagon to patients for rather a long time.

Jaspan: Professor Paul has used glucagon for two weeks, and we have used it for three, and found it to be perfectly safe. As far as a possible diabetogenic risk is concerned, Liljenquist and Cherrington and their group in Nashville, and Felig, have provided evidence that even though hyperglycaemia occurs initially with glucagon infusion, the blood sugar levels subsequently fall towards normal. This effect has been termed 'down-regulation'. (Bombay, J.D. Jr. *et al.* (1977), *Diabetes,* **26,** 177; Bloomgarden, Z.T. *et al.* (1978). *J. Clin. Endocrin. Metab.,* **47,** 1152; Felig, P. *et al.* (1976), *Diabetes,* **25,** 1091; Shulman, G.I. *et al.* (1977), *Diabetes,* **26,** suppl. 1, 383). There is not a great effect, therefore, on blood sugar levels with glucagon infusion in non-diabetics, and when given with insulin infusion, as we have done in our studies, this small effect is minimized. As far as diabetes is concerned, I agree with other speakers here that it should certainly not be regarded as a contraindication for glucagon. One has simply to adjust the experience of the cardiologists, and now of the gastroenterologists, the radiologists, and the endoscopists, as well as our own findings, I would say that glucagon appears to be one of the safest drugs available today.

Paul: One word of caution: I would hesitate to use glucagon in cases with juvenile brittle diabetes. If one has had difficulties stabilizing a patient on insulin, and when alternative solutions are available, it would be unwise to change the insulin regimen and risk the problems starting all over again. Such cases are rare, however. As far as other diabetics are concerned, I would foresee no difficulties. We have infused glucagon in diabetics for 8–10 days with no problems at all.

Jaspan: Regarding deleterious effects of glucagon, Gerich and co-workers have shown that when insulin is withdrawn from diabetics in whom somatostatin has been used to suppress glucagon the onset of ketosis could be delayed (Gerich, J.E. *et al.* (1975), *N. Engl. J. Med.,* **292,** 985.

Clarke *et al.* (1978, *Diabetes,* **27,** 649) have studied the effect of hyperglucagonaemia on blood glucose concentrations and on insulin requirements in insulin-requiring diabetes. Hyperglucagonaemia was induced by means of constant intravenous infusion. Raising the glucagon levels to around 500 pg/ml did not alter total insulin requirements or blood sugar levels. When raised to levels of around 1000 pg/ml there was a small increase in insulin requirements with only minimal increases in blood sugar levels. Accordingly, in diabetics who are on insulin there.appear to be no adverse effects of glucagon administration, although if large amounts of glucagon were to be given over a period of time a small increase in insulin dose may be required.

Chairman: What about the hepatotrophic effects?

Volpicelli: The only therapeutic experience with glucagon so far has been in mice. Frankly, I would be afraid to try the levels used in mice in humans, as this would mean doses of approximately 1.5 mg glucagon per hour to a person weighing 50 kg. The doses we plan to give in our study are 3 mg per day for a 50 kg patient, which is about the same as those used by Professor Paul, and a little higher than those being used in the Chicago study. This should give us levels of 8000–10 000 pg/ml of serum, which is approaching the levels seen in patients with glucagonoma. We are expecting to encounter some problems – the ones usually seen in patients with glucagonoma – but not insurmountable ones.

Chairman: At this point, the scheduled finishing time being long passed, this discussion session had to be closed, though, as can be imagined, the talking continued into the night.

The consensus of opinion of those taking part, hard-pressed though we were to cover so much ground in just one day, was that this workshop was an extremely valuable and stimulating one.

It is hoped that in the papers presented, you, the reader, will find much of interest and help, and that in the edited discussions you will find that at least some of the points which you yourself would have wished to raise were in fact satisfactorily covered. The addresses of the people taking part in this workshop are given at the front of this book, and I hope that you will not hesitate to contact these people should you have questions to ask, opinions to express, or experiences to relate, for in this way the debate so interestingly begun at this workshop can be continued.

Index